TRAINING FOR LIFE

TRAINING FOR LIFE

Walk Your Way to Fitness and Weight Loss in 14 Days

DEBBIE ROCKER

with LAURA TUCKER

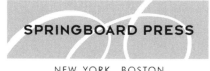

SPRINGBOARD PRESS

NEW YORK   BOSTON

Springboard Press
Hachette Book Group USA
237 Park Avenue, New York, NY 10169
Visit our Web site at www.HachetteBookGroupUSA.com

Springboard Press is an imprint of Warner Books. The Springboard name
and logo are trademarks of Hachette Book Group USA.

First Edition: April 2007

Library of Congress Cataloging-in-Publication Data

Rocker, Debbie.
    Training for life: walk your way to fitness and weight loss in 14 days /
Debbie Rocker — 1st ed.
       p. cm.
ISBN 978-0-446-58102-8
1. Fitness walking. 2. Physical fitness. 3. Walking — Health aspects.
4. Weight loss. I. Title.

RA781.65.R64 2006
613.7′176 — dc22   2006002578

10 9 8 7 6 5 4 3 2 1

Q-FF

Book design by Jo Anne Metsch

Printed in the United States of America

Dedication

I am guided and supported by *well-being*, the Divine nature of the Universe, and I thank God that I know that.

To my family: You have each given me (probably without even knowing it) something so loving, so valuable, and so permanent. Each one of you has impressed upon me, in your own special way, how important it is for us to be genuinely ourselves. I love you all.

Hirsh: Your spirit in business, and in life, is the same: generous, hopeful, and endlessly confident. But more important still is our friendship: I have always, always, always needed a friend like you.

Tory: You have seen me, really known me, and still trusted and believed in me. You have tirelessly and lovingly helped me help myself, and I thank you for your unwavering faith in and unconditional love for me.

Nina: You have helped me feel whole, healthy, and complete. You have been gentle, generous, kind beyond reason, and a springboard for moving forward in my life.

Training for Life is dedicated to all of you.

Contents

PART TWO: TRAINING FOR LIFE: THE PROGRAM

PART THREE: LIVING YOUR TRAINING

Acknowledgments

Many people participated in the creation of this book, and I would like to thank all of them, particularly:

Carol Mann: My literary agent. Wow, it just occurred to me that I have an agent — but not just an agent, a special person who trusted me, and my instincts, and helped me realize a dream. Thank you.

Jill Cohen and Karen Murgolo: My publisher and my editor. We had an immediate respect for, and understanding of, each other's needs and desires, and had a shared vision that grew into a relationship and a book. What a pleasure. To you who graciously and generously opened the gates of opportunity for me — please accept my heartfelt respect and thanks.

This book, too, is for you.

Laura Tucker: My collaborator and co-writer. I really cannot thank you enough! Your insight, intelligence, and professionalism made writing this book a pleasure. Your enthusiasm and ability to embrace my ideas, your understanding of me and of my way of seeing things as we progressed made our partnership a rewarding and joyful one. I send great thanks and appreciation to you.

— Debbie Rocker

First and foremost I'd like to thank the amazing Debbie Rocker. Her wisdom and sense of humor made this collaboration a truly wonderful experience.

I'd also like to thank the following people: Carol Mann for the introduction and her assistance along the way; Jill Cohen, Jamie Raab, Karen Murgolo, and the team at Springboard for their tireless support; the Tuckers, the Crowells, and Latoya Kelly for pinch-hitting; and Doug and Lily for everything else.

— *Laura Tucker*

Preface

We're out of shape for our lives.

Molly still blames "baby weight" for the forty extra pounds she's carrying on her petite frame, although her youngest child is eight. She hates full-length mirrors and won't let her husband see her without clothes; needless to say, the romance in that relationship is dwindling.

Jane has spent the last fifteen years losing and then gaining back the same twenty-five pounds. By now she has two complete wardrobes: a fat one and a skinny one — and two personalities to match.

Donna looks great, but maintaining her beautiful body is driving her — and everyone around her — crazy. She hasn't eaten butter or a whole egg since nonfat foods got their own aisle in the supermarket, and at restaurants she makes waiters and everyone else at the table miserable with her list of demands. On one memorable occasion she ignored the menu entirely and ate carrots from a Tupperware container with the restaurant's silverware.

Alex's doctor has read him the riot act over his high cholesterol. Alex knows he's in trouble; he can barely breathe when he climbs the short flight of stairs up to his office door, and he hates what he sees in the mirror. But he says that no matter what he does, he can't seem to shed the pounds that are killing him.

Almost everyone I know is out of shape, and not just physically. More and more, striving for the so-called American Dream is turning our lives into nightmares. We're overworked and unfulfilled, undernourished and overfed, quick-tempered and slowly running ourselves into the ground. Obesity is at an all-time high, and so is the money we're pouring into the diet and weight-loss industry.

I'm here to tell you that you can stop that cycle right now, if you want to. You can stop wasting your precious resources — your money, your time, your energy, and your life — searching for "a cure" for being overweight. Whether you've struggled with weight issues your whole life or are finding that you now have to be more vigilant about what you put into your mouth, you can improve your state of health and fitness. Whether you're someone who's never set foot in a gym or someone whose regular work-outs need a good shaking-up, I guarantee that you will benefit enormously from this program. In fact I guarantee that if you give me fourteen days, I will get you off the "diet-go-round," improving your body and your state of mind — for good.

My program and coaching will radically change how your body looks in fourteen days or less, but that's not all. This program is about how you look and how you feel, what you believe about yourself, and how you act. Over the next two weeks, you and I together will build the foundation you need for fundamental changes that last a life-time. You will work out hard enough to feel your body, and you will become quiet enough to hear your inner voice. As you become stronger, healthier, and more self-aware, you will be able to transform your life, *which includes losing weight for good.* For the first time you will be training for **total fitness** — mind and body fitness — and you will have the tools to make those changes permanent.

From this moment on you're an athlete in training for the longest, most challenging, and most important event that any one of us will ever enter. From this moment on, you are in *Training for Life*.

PART ONE

THE ROAD AHEAD

CHAPTER 1

Diagnosis: Dis-ease

"I'm eating all the wrong stuff," Jane tells me sheepishly. "I have got to get back on my diet; South Beach is the only thing that ever worked for me."

I answer her as gently as I can: "Jane, if South Beach really 'worked' for you, it would *still be working*."

I know that Jane lost lots of weight the last time she "did" South Beach, and I'm sure that some of the other blockbuster diets she's tried have worked too — but for whatever reason, those changes are never permanent for her. Like most of us Jane eats not because she's hungry, but because she's starving — for something that food cannot give her. It's not a need for physical nourishment that drives her to the refrigerator, but a need for a reward, or for comfort, or for love. Like Jane, many of us are confused, tired, lonely, bored, overwhelmed, marginalized. Like her, many of us temporarily "fix" ourselves with food. And we all pay a very high price for that temporary comfort in self-loathing, in poor self-esteem, and in the health risks we assume by being overweight.

The worst part of all is that when we bury our feelings under a box of cookies, we never do the work necessary to satisfy our true hungers. If you're overweight there's a very good chance that you're romantically, socially, financially, emotionally, or intellectually famished. But Jane truly believes her weight problem is physical, so she contributes generously to the billions of dollars spent every year by Americans on weight-loss tapes, diet books, gym memberships, exercise equipment, magic flab-melting supplements, and low-carb, low-calorie, low-fat foods.

And it works — for a while. Every New Year, Jane swears off booze and sugar, starts walking in the morning before work and drinking more water, and lo and behold, she drops a few pounds and feels a little better about herself.

But Jane's new regimen doesn't represent an essential, fundamental, meaningful change; all she's done is temporarily replace eating with dieting and exercise. All her fears and anxieties, the things that really make her want to eat, are just lying in wait. When they pounce — and they always do — she watches the needle inch ever higher on the scale as the weight she lost finds her again, and the pounds reaccumulate on her frame. She feels terrible about herself, not just because she's back to her "fat" jeans, but because she lost another battle with herself.

My purpose is to get you — and Jane and Molly and Donna and Alex — working with, instead of against, yourself. To do that I must make some radical requests of you, starting with this one: take all of the diet and fitness lore you've been collecting from magazines and daytime TV shows, Web sites, your friends, and variously appointed nutrition and fitness gurus, stick it in a box, and forget about it for fourteen days. If at the end of those fourteen days you don't feel a very positive change in yourself, you can throw this book in the trash and go back to whatever you were doing (or *not* doing) before.

I'm not saying that all that diet and fitness information out there is bad. The problem is that there isn't a magic formula. Of course it's a good idea to choose whole carbohydrates over refined ones or to eat more lightly at night. But the idea that your whole weight-loss puzzle will snap into place when you find just the right piece of diet and exercise trivia — Do cardio after your strength training! Don't eat tomatoes on the same day you eat blueberries! — is a way of thinking about our weight and our health that gets us into trouble. Go sugar free, nonfat, dairy free, wheat free; eat all the steak and eggs you can stomach, they tell us. But these are fads; they don't represent a way of life. All they do is keep the diet industry booming and you on the weight-loss seesaw. Let me give you the power to get off — and to stay off.

It's not that there isn't an equation for healthy weight loss. There *is:*

Eat less and be more active.

But you know that already. And if losing weight was really that simple, we wouldn't be a nation of desperate and overweight people dumping billions of dollars every year into the diet industry. So where's the disconnect? If we have the key, why can't we open the door?

The truth is that while many diets work, they don't work *permanently*. Why? Because they ignore the biggest contributor to our long-term success: our minds. You know that you have to train your body to change; doesn't it make sense that you'd have to train your mind as well? Results that last a lifetime are attainable only by making your mind as healthy as your body.

True fitness isn't simply physical.

Our thoughts, feelings, beliefs, fears, and obsessions drive our actions and behaviors. Unless we deal with our weight problems at the mind-body intersection, the self-destructive cycle continues: short-term weight loss followed by even more weight gain and even more negative, shameful feelings about ourselves.

So for this short period of time, you have to take a leap of faith. I am asking you — even if it's just for these fourteen days — to let go of all those diet dos and don'ts and trust me. Do something different this time and let go of the belief that there's some magic that will effortlessly transform your body. Unless you surrender that belief, you will get in your way and mine. In exchange for your brave efforts, I will give you back the very thing that has eluded you for all these years: a fit body and peace of mind.

You won't be alone, either; I know how hard it is to change. We all need help, and that's where I come in.

Effective training tools are important, but *coaching is imperative* to reaching new levels of fitness.

A good coach can take you places you can't go alone. I've spent the majority of my adult life working and playing with fitness for body and mind. As a professional coach and motivator, I know what it will take to bring out the best in you; as a former pro athlete, I know what will work. We're starting from scratch, working from the ground up, and I will be with you, every single step of the way.

As you strengthen your muscles, you'll realize that this new strength goes far deeper than just physical strength. You're going to shed bad habits as you shed the excess weight, and you'll reshape your body as you realign your thinking.

Ultimately a new you will appear, and that "new you" will be not only stronger and leaner but also more confident and *happier,* too. This is because being overweight is just a symptom of your "dis-ease." The same fears and insecurities that make you overeat are also behind your uneasy relationships with your children, your dissatisfaction with your salary, the sneaking suspicion that your sex life isn't as fabulous as it could be. In a way you should be grateful to those excess pounds — they've brought you to this place of change.

In your effort to lose the excess weight, you're going to change *every single area* of your life for the better.

And because your training will not only create but support your beliefs and behaviors, you can be confident that this new you will not only survive for a short time but thrive for a lifetime. Let me guide, coach, motivate, and empower you so that you can get into shape — great shape — for your great life.

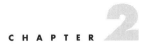

Total Conditioning: A Mind-Body Solution to a Mind-Body Problem

"Action seems to follow feeling, but really action and feeling go together; and by regulating the action, which is under the more direct control of the will, we can indirectly regulate the feeling, which is not."

—WILLIAM JAMES

True fitness isn't just physical. Training for Life will get your body into dramatically better shape, but the physical changes will be just a small part of a much bigger transformation. Our real goal together is something bigger: total fitness.

Total fitness is an entirely new way of thinking about the concept of fitness. It's not just about getting thinner, and it's certainly not about doing it short term. Total fitness is about getting healthier and stronger, for the long haul. And it's not just about your body. Total fitness will get your mind and spirit strong and healthy, too, and give you the self-respect, self-acceptance, and self-appreciation that comes from knowing you can achieve whatever goals you set for yourself.

In other words, total fitness means getting *every part of you* in shape — your body and your mind — so you're in prime condition to live the life you want and deserve.

Another Way of Looking at the Problem

When you think about your life, and the things about it you'd like to change, I'll bet there's more than just "pant size" on the list. Like many of my students, you probably feel stuck in many different areas of your life. Sure, you're uncomfortable with your weight — but also with your job, your relationships, your income, and other things, too.

In fact your struggle with your weight is just one manifestation of a much larger issue: your struggle with yourself. And so is your discomfort in your job, with your marriage, or with your paycheck. All the different parts of you — who you are and what you do — are related. To get to a better place, not just physically, but in all these areas, you'll have to deal with that bigger struggle. But the quick-fix diets and the miraculous weight-loss machines and potions "as seen on" late-night television ignore everything we know about the powerful mind-body connection. They suggest that you should address your weight problems exclusively through diet and exercise, as if these issues were separate from the rest of your life. They're trying to tell you — and sell you — the idea that there is a body-only solution to what is clearly a mind-and-body problem.

You already know that Training for Life means throwing out a lot of stale beliefs and misconceptions. I'd like this particular misconception — the preposterous idea that our bodies and our minds are separate — to be one of the first ones you throw overboard. In this chapter I'll show you how this misconception sets you up to fail at dieting and supports the diet roller coaster you've been on.

The struggle with our waistlines is a serious problem, and one that I can help you put behind you forever, but I believe it is symptomatic of a greater malaise. I believe we'd struggle a whole lot less with our outer, physical selves — not to mention our bosses, our kids, and our spending practices — if we really focused on developing our sense of awareness, responsibility, and compassion for our inner selves and for those around us. That's why the training in Training for Life focuses as much on what's going on *inside* as it does on your physical body.

An Unconscious Life

Most of us live on autopilot. We are creatures of habit, programmed according to our past conditioning. We eat dinner every night at six o'clock, whether we're hungry or not, and have dessert whether we're full or not, because that's what we've always done. As kids we were rewarded with delicious goodies, bribed to stop crying with edible treats, and punished by having the sweets taken away. So now the Hershey bar we once got for a good report card has turned into a box of Godiva to celebrate a big deal, and the cookie we got to console us for getting picked last for the team has turned into a pint of ice cream after a fight with a lover.

We've continued to eat (and drink) instead of feeling our feelings. We've treated our disappointments with a junk-food pity party in front of the TV and our self-hatred with an extra piece of lasagna. We're grown-ups now, but food (or its many substitutes: a few too many glasses of wine, charges to a credit-card bill we know we can't afford) is still the reward, the consolation prize, and the punishment, all rolled into one. The problem is that now we're completely out of touch with the feelings that are causing us to eat and drink. Without that information we're helpless to break the cycle: feeling, eating, dieting, cheating, feeling, eating, dieting, cheating. . . .

As odd as it may seem, that excess weight serves us in some important way, although we'll swear up and down that we hate it, especially when bathing-suit season rolls around. Many of us use the extra padding as a buffer to protect us from the feelings that make us uncomfortable: loneliness, self-doubt, inadequacy — and our fear of success, too.

Truly, you wouldn't put your whole life in such discomfort if you knew deep down that feelings are only temporary and harmless. But our feelings do feel fatal, and not understanding what they are or what they mean makes us feel out of control — and there's *nothing* we hate more than being out of control. There is one thing that we *can* control, and that is keeping the weight on; we seem to know how to do that, without even trying. So although we don't control the weather, what people think of us, or what we feel, we *can* make ourselves overweight and use that to insulate ourselves from failure and success. We can use it to stay in the same, stuck place, confirming what we've been told (and now tell ourselves): that we're not capable, or deserving, of a better life.

Clearly the way out of this conundrum is to begin to address these feelings, which are the root causes of our self-destructive behavior. Traditional diet programs don't — and that's one of the main reasons they'll all eventually fail you.

The Chain of Command

Traditional diets support yet another dangerous fallacy. They tell you that working out will make you look and feel terrific. That's true — but they also say that looking and feeling great will be all the incentive you need to keep going forever. The problem? That's not how human beings work.

Most of us can follow a diet or workout program for a while, especially when we're losing weight and looking good. So why doesn't it ever last? Why is it just a matter of time before we start cheating or treating and eating again? Why isn't looking and feeling good from the weight loss enough to keep us on track?

Because you haven't made any fundamental changes to your mind. So all your new behaviors are actually running contrary to your deep-seated beliefs about who you are, what you're capable of, and what you deserve. What we see with our "inner eye" is what we believe about ourselves, so that vision of ourselves is as important as (if not more important than) what we see in the mirror. If you haven't changed your beliefs or the way the current of information flows in your mind, your results won't last. Nobody can keep swimming against the tide without becoming exhausted; inevitably you will give up and go back to behaving self-destructively in order to be consistent with your fundamental belief that you don't deserve anything better.

I know people who have undergone gastric bypass surgery and lost tremendous amounts of weight; I am sure you have read their stories as well. One magazine wrote about a woman who, after surgery and great weight loss, walked right into a mirror — she no longer recognized her own image! This is a dramatic example of what happens when the body changes and the mind fails to accommodate the change, and as far as I'm concerned, it doesn't bode well for this particular woman's long-term success. It's very uncomfortable to live with that kind of dissonance between body and mind, and I wouldn't want to bet on a contest between the brain, the most powerful supercomputer on earth, and a few stomach staples.

You may believe that losing weight will improve your self-esteem and silence the negative monologue you hear in your head. But losing weight will fix your weight problem; to fix your self-esteem, we have to address your self-esteem. And that's the key to keeping the weight off for good. If you don't get your mind in shape at the same time as you improve your body, your mind is going to drag you right back to where you started.

There is no surgery for changing our minds, our beliefs, and what we see when we look at ourselves with our inner eye. But there are simple conditioning exercises that you can do to gradually encourage your mind to accept and support your new lifestyle.

**Reconditioning yourself — body and mind — is the key
to your long-term weight loss and total fitness goals.**

Training for Life is not a more difficult process than anything you've done in the past, but it *does* require that you recognize the real chain of command. The mind doesn't follow the body; the body follows the mind. Your thoughts and beliefs create and support your behaviors, *not* the other way around.

If you're reading this book, you've undoubtedly tried to lose weight a number of times and failed — or you've succeeded and then failed. In the process you have further conditioned yourself to fail at weight loss — providing you with a new insecurity, which stacks on top of all the other, deep-seated ones.

It's time to break the cycle. I am here, and Training for Life is here, to bring YOU powerfully back in charge of your life. There are three really good reasons to embrace total — mind-body — fitness.

First of all, the physical results will come easier, since the mental conditioning will help you to make the choices that get you the results you want quickly. Second, conditioning and changing our minds is completely essential for *maintaining* weight loss. This is especially true when life gets tough, and it's easy to slip back into the old, self-destructive ways of coping — like eating to soothe yourself. Staying strong and staying slim through the ups and downs that your life will inevitably present over the years depends much more on your mental state than on your physical one. Last, and maybe most important, when you learn how to really change your life, not just your body, you will have a set of magnificent tools that you can use to become unstuck in every other area of your life, too — not just your weight.

We'll do this with some counterconditioning practices for our minds combined with effective conditioning exercises for our bodies. Add a little common sense, some self-discipline, your pure efforts, and some proven motivational coaching, and you have an equation that is sure to change *more* than just your body, and for more than just a few weeks.

How Training for Life Gives You Total Fitness

To train for life you have to train your mind as well as your body — you have to work out, and you have to work *in*. Your mind guides your actions; that's why I call this mental conditioning "Training Your Trainer" and why you'll find notes from me to your "Inner Coach" throughout this book. I have designed this book and my CDs so that you'll always be able to return to my coaching, but the goal of this program is to make you not dependent on me but able to rely on yourself for all the direction and motivation you need to keep going.

Ultimately only *you* can determine whether you're going to get out of bed on a cold morning to work out or roll over for another hour of sleep. You are the only one who can decide if you're going to reach for another cookie or for a piece of fruit. You are the one who will decide whether it's worth it to make the effort to be the best you can possibly be. So as you train your body, you're going to be training your Inner Coach as well.

Let me explain how this works. During your Training for Life **WorkOuts** you will burn calories and fat, strengthen your heart and lungs, build lean muscle and bone density, and tone and sculpt your body. Each WorkOut, incidentally, will be perfectly calibrated to your personal level of fitness. Each will require you to give a significant physical effort, but one appropriately fit to you. Your WorkOuts will be safe, effective, interesting, and motivational, and though you'll feel their effects immediately, they won't hurt you, and you won't dread doing one the next day — in fact you may even look forward to it!

But that's just half of the Training for Life program. The second part involves exercising, conditioning, and changing your mind, and that's where a series of mental exercises called **WorkIns** come in. These WorkIns are mind-conditioning exercises that will isolate and eliminate self-destructive behaviors at their root. They'll help you to form positive beliefs about who you are, what you're capable of, and what you deserve in your life. With these simple, repetitive, empowering exercises, we can rewire your thinking so that you no longer sabotage your victories or inhibit your own success. These exercises are what have been missing in your previous efforts, and they are the foundation for permanent change.

Your body needs repetitious conditioning to change, and so does your mind.

Every day I will give you a WorkIn with a phrase to take away with you and repeat over and over to yourself. You will say it as many times as you can remember to, with a minimum of twenty-four times a day. Different cultures have different names for a practice like this, including meditation, prayer, or repeating a mantra. They have been utilized and followed for thousands and thousands of years because they work, and as you probably already know, they are making their way back into popular culture because they are so effective.

You might think the WorkIns are hocus-pocus, and you may feel silly doing them. You may be asked to repeat words that sound corny to you or "unlike you," contrary to who you believe you are. I felt the same way — before these practices changed my life. No matter how you feel about them, you should know that these WorkIns are critical and are at the core of my program; without them, any transformation will be only skin-deep.

So you'll do your WorkIns as you get dressed in the morning, drive to work, prepare dinner — and especially while you work out. Why? When we are physically engaged, we achieve a state of being more sensitive and receptive than usual. You may have noticed that you sometimes feel "high" or very emotional during a workout. Exercising releases natural chemicals in our bodies. These can help to break down the barriers we ordinarily use to protect ourselves from our feelings. I have always said that one-on-one fitness trainers and group exercise instructors have a great responsibility because of the hypersensitive, receptive state their clients may be in. It's a great time to provide useful and positive messages, though, and that's what we'll do as we train for life.

As you work out, you will reflect on the day's WorkIn. As your muscles warm up, becoming more limber and malleable, so will your mind. As you get deeper into your WorkOut, you'll find that it is easier to make caring and positive statements about yourself and to believe them. Soon your WorkIn will become more personal, taking on a meaning just for you. In this way the practices of working out and working in facilitate and support each other, for faster and more long-lasting results.

It's time to put these techniques to work for you. You have agreed to throw out the old and give the new a try. This particular new practice, one that you do in the privacy of your mind, must be done with the commit-

ROCKER'S RULES OF TOTAL FITNESS

- Your health and your happiness depend on the fitness of your body and your mind.

- You create your fitness.

- You can change your fitness.

- Total fitness is a mind and body proposition.

- Total fitness is the key to permanent fitness.

ment and conviction of a prizefighter. It will help you to bring your head and heart together in a comfortable union, so that your results can easily stay forever.

A New Age of Awareness

Ultimately what Training for Life will do is bring you a new level of awareness.

We sabotage ourselves, both consciously and unconsciously. We "taste" a whole dinner's worth of food while we're cooking; we grab a few chocolates from the bowl every time we pass; we look up at the end of a sitcom to realize that we've eaten the whole bag. Even when we can predict what the unfortunate consequences of our actions will be, we still find ourselves following the same worn grooves of our old habits, as if we had no choice in the matter at all.

You do have a choice, and awareness gives you the chance to make it. First, it pulls back the covers, so you can no longer live in denial. If you didn't know you were eating an extra thousand calories a day, now you will. And with awareness, you create space between thought and action, so that you can choose to put your kid's leftover grilled cheese into the trash instead of your mouth. Ultimately you'll be able to hear what your body needs — as well as what doesn't work for it — and that's information that you can use to protect and improve it, keeping it youthful and powerful for as long as you possibly can.

I'd like to emphasize that awareness *doesn't* mean giving up the things that you love to eat. That's a traditional diet trap — of course you'll keep losing weight as long as you pledge never to have another bite of birthday cake! But that's not realistic, and it isn't the kind of glorious life I'm training you for.

I remember a new friend expressing incredulity when I ordered a piece of homemade peach pie at my favorite restaurant after lunch together. "I wouldn't have guessed you'd order dessert," she said. It's true — I usually don't. But that's why I can, every once in a while. If you're ordering a piece of pie because you want it and because you will enjoy it, then it won't derail you. It's when you order one every night, or sit down with the whole pie, or eat it and feel self-destructive that it causes harm.

When you Train for Life, the perfect piece of pie isn't even "off message"; it's one healthy, responsible choice among the many you make that are taking you toward your goal of being slim and fit, happy and healthy. You don't have to feel bad about it, because you've made it with awareness, and it fits in with all the other responsible, healthy choices you make.

The mental and physical training techniques in this program are specifically designed to help you gain this new awareness quickly so that you can make significant changes in your body, and your life, and continue to support those important modifications with healthy, mindful choices.

After you've done a few of the WorkOuts and WorkIns, you'll begin to notice a change, as your mind and body begin to sync up with one another. And you'll find that this new awareness will unlock the door to a lot of places you've spent a long time trying to get into. The answer to the question "Isn't there anything more to life than this?" is yes, yes, yes. There's happiness, pride, productivity, and contentment. There is much more, and now you can choose it. There is love, vitality, personal enhancement, and joy. You can have it all, if you choose to, and I absolutely feel that you deserve to.

By buying this book you have certainly taken the first step toward changing your body — but let's not stop there. Let's work together and use awareness to bring your mind in line with your body, your thinking in line with your actions, and your desires in line with your choices so that you're as efficient, powerful, and happy in your life as you can be.

CHAPTER 3

Walking: The Body's Most Natural Form of Exercise

One of the reasons Training for Life works so well for so many people is that it uses walking as the primary form of physical exercise.

The "no pain, no gain" philosophy of the last thirty years may have made orthopedists rich, but it failed the rest of us. Instead of effectively improving our bodies, the exercises that were recommended put us in harm's way and pushed many of us to the point of injury. We were looking for a fitness program that we could seamlessly incorporate into our lives, but the ones out there gave too many of us the impression that what we *could* do wasn't enough, so we hung up our sneakers for good.

What you'll find in Training for Life is very different. After all, this program grew out of what I have always wanted for my students, and for myself. What do I want? I want a workout that will give me a lean, toned, strong body, a youthful appearance, and great health — without taking energy away from the rest of my life. The workouts must be comprehensive — as good for my muscles and bones as they are for my heart and lungs — so that I'm getting the most for my exercise time, while still being compassionate to my body. And I don't want to be tied to a trainer, instructor, membership, or major financial commitment.

Impossible, you might be thinking. But the answer is right in front of you. In fact the most healthful, inexpensive, and effective exercise on earth is something that our ancestors spent the last 200,000 years perfecting and something that you've done almost every day of your life: the two-legged walk.

Simply put, walking is *the healthiest and most natural* exercise for your body.

Human beings are designed to walk.

That's why just about everyone can do it, regardless of age, exercise experience, or their current level of physical fitness. Walking for fitness is *right* for everybody. I know: my students run the gamut. They range from well-conditioned professional athletes to grandparents in their eighties. I have trained full-time fashion models, brand-new moms, burly law-enforcement officers, weekend warriors, and men and women working to recover their strength after chemotherapy treatments — and every single one of them walks for fitness, with great results. And I'm in there, too — this isn't something that I read about or saw on TV; it's how I got to be the fittest, leanest, and most energetic I've ever been in my life. But more about me later. . . .

Overcoming Diminishing Returns

Of course the fact that we're designed to walk can be both a blessing and a curse. You see, our bodies adapt to carrying our natural weight, as we naturally adapt to anything, including any exercise that we do over a period of time. That adaptation leads to diminishing returns — although we're doing the same amount of exercise, we're not seeing the same results we used to.

One solution is to exercise harder, and for longer periods of time, but that's not very efficient: pushing ourselves will make exercise less pleasurable, and who has more time to devote to it? My strategy is to *work more effectively*. You can do that by adding professional guidance and new programming to maximize your exercise time. And adding weight, or resistance, helps to overcome the body's natural adaptations, so you're not doing more, but you get more.

My training system does both. You'll always have the benefit of my coaching in this book and on CD, and I've developed an adjustable weight-loaded vest called WalkVest that transforms ordinary walking into a highly effective workout without altering your natural stride or hurting your back, like hand and ankle weights can do.

Here's why my walking workouts — with or without a WalkVest — are so transformative:

· **They work!** Done properly, walking is an incredibly powerful, cardio-strengthening, calorie-burning, fat-melting form of exercise. *Prevention* magazine has said that "there is no easier way to lose weight than walking," and the Mayo Clinic asserts that "brisk walking burns as many calories as running that same distance." Add a weighted vest, and the results increase exponentially.

I like to call my walking workouts (whether you're wearing a WalkVest while doing them or not) WalkOuts because they offer more comprehensive, total body conditioning than any walking you've ever done before. Trust me, this isn't your grandmother's walk around the block.

· **They're safe.** Doctors, surgeons, and chiropractors feel confident recommending walking (and walking in the WalkVest) for losing weight, gaining strength, increasing cardiovascular endurance, and building bone density — without injury or pain.

Consulting with your physician before engaging in any new exercise or diet plan is always a good idea; in this case I'll bet he or she not only signs off on Training for Life but tells you it's the best thing you've ever done for yourself.

· **They come with your own personal coach.** No matter how resistant you are, I know that motivational coaching can get you to work out, enjoy it, and get lasting results. And when you have a coach guiding and encouraging you, the benefits of your training will increase dramatically. You'll become fitter faster and inspired to stay that way because of the power of total fitness, which trains your mind as well as your body. You'll find that when you work with a coach to condition yourself, mentally and physically, there's nothing you can't do.

Every WalkOut includes coaching, so you can read what you'd hear if I were walking right next to you, and it's why I've included a CD with this book. Every WalkVest comes with motivational coaching and music on CD as well.

· **You can do these WorkOuts with others.** Walking is one of those exercises that actually gets better with a partner or in a group, so put some fun back into your workouts by getting social.

Walking with others will help you to mix it up so you don't get bored, and knowing that someone is out there waiting for you adds an extra layer of accountability. Training for Life makes it easy to be social by varying the intensity and duration of your training days. A recovery day WalkOut, which is less intense, gives you the perfect opportunity to work out with a friend. If you choose to team up with a TFL buddy on a more intense day, just be sure the company doesn't distract you from the task at hand!

I'm pleased to report that WalkVest walking groups have sprung up around the country; I've walked with some of them, and I can see why they're so popular. It makes daily exercise fun and can be extremely motivating, as the power of the group inspires those in it to reach beyond their own individual limits.

Many of the group members report that they've developed very meaningful relationships as well. I had the privilege of walking with a group called the Shoreham Walk-Vesters, in Shoreham, New York. They meet every morning at six a.m., rain or shine, to walk and talk or to listen to one of my CDs. Everyone in town knows them, and no one passes without a honk of support or a few words of encouragement. The women in the group have also bonded tightly as a unit. Together they have discarded the clothing that has grown too big for them and the ideas that grew too small.

Since the WalkVest weight is adjustable, people of varying fitness levels can effectively WalkOut together. I walk with my mom; she wears four pounds in her vest, while I wear eight, and we both are getting great workouts, appropriate to our own fitness levels, while we spend some quality time together.

These WorkOuts can be done as easily as stepping out your front door. With or without a WalkVest, you can *always* walk: wherever you live or travel to, no matter the terrain or climate. You can do your WalkOuts on your lunch break, on vacation, or on a business trip. You can hike in the great outdoors, trek the urban jungle, or walk at the mall, as millions of Americans already do.

You may even decide, as I do, to wear your WalkVest while walking your dogs, cleaning up after the kids, and running errands — I never leave home without mine. My students walk in the morning before work, at night after the kids are in bed, and even on their way to work. They'll park twenty blocks away from the commuter train or their office or get off the subway two stops before their destination. Those miles add up by week's end!

IT TAKES A VILLAGE

People who have been successful in losing weight and keeping it off have a few things in common. One is that they exercise. The other is that they have support: families who agree to keep cookies and chips out of the cupboards, friends to swap healthy recipes with and to share their victories with.

Many successful "losers" have a group to weigh in with; exercise buddies that they have a commitment to; and a coach, mentor, or program that gives them guidelines for their practice. So if you've ever thought, "I can't do this alone," you're probably right. The good news is that you don't have to. First of all you have me and this book, the *Training for Life* manual, and I'll bet that when you start asking around, you'll find that you're not the only person who wants to start training for a better life.

The TFL WalkOuts build bone density. We all lose bone density as we age, beginning as early as age thirty. If we don't take measures to counteract this loss through weight-bearing exercise, bone loss can turn into osteoporosis, a disease that leaves bones porous and fragile, so that they break easily and heal slowly. More than 10 million Americans are afflicted with osteoporosis; most of them are women.

Osteoporosis often goes undetected until it is too late — with horrifying consequences. The disease causes 1.5 million fractures each year, and in over 300,000 of those cases, it leads to death; another 1.2 million people will require long-term nursing care because of complications. It is a devastating disease — perhaps even more so because it is *preventable and reversible.*

A staggering 34 million Americans have a condition called osteopenia, or low bone mass. This is a precursor to osteoporosis. Doctors typically recommend walking as a weight-bearing exercise to help prevent further bone loss, especially in the lower body, but it may not be enough. I hear this frequently: "My doctor told me to walk to build bone mass, and I do — five days a week! — but she still wants to put me on bone-building medications to prevent full-blown osteoporosis. What am I doing wrong?" You're not doing *anything* wrong; although you are walking on a regular basis, you're simply running up against your body's natural adaptation to the exercise, so you're not getting adequate weight-bearing benefits.

What's the alternative? Well, you can take up jogging or start jumping rope; those activities can help to build bone mass. But they're potentially damaging in other ways and not something that most of us can do joyfully — or consistently. There's a better, more effective, and safer solution: walking with added weight, or *resistance.*

Dr. Christine Snow, the head of the Bone Research Laboratory at Oregon State University, has demonstrated in numerous studies that exercising in a weighted vest is ideal for people with reduced bone mass. This type of exercise prevents further bone loss, increases actual bone strength and density, and reverses the losses already suffered. There's an added bonus as well: walking with a weighted vest also strengthens connective tissues. This strengthens and secures the body's most fundamental structure — our skeleton — as well as helping with posture and balance, which minimizes the risk of falling, the leading cause of those fatal fractures. Adding a WalkVest to your WalkOuts, as Dr. Snow's patients do, will combat the insidious creep of bone loss and increase bone density and improve fitness in other ways, too.

If you want to find out more about WalkVest, or how to buy one, go to my Web site: www.walkvest.com.

Total Body Fitness

In the same way that we're going to give a great deal of thought and attention to the balance between our bodies and minds, it's essential for our physical conditioning to reflect a good balance.

In order to achieve that balance, we must effectively condition both our upper and lower bodies, as well as our core. We must exercise for *strength*, or muscle power, as well as for *endurance*, or staying power. Our priorities must be equally divided between appearance — weight control, our posture, and the tone of our muscles — and essential functioning, like making our hearts, lungs, bones, and the muscles that support them strong. We'll do all this, and once in a while, we'll even rest!

Walking, naturally (and thankfully) targets our legs and rear end. Since that's where most of the work takes place, that's where you'll see results first. Whether you choose to do the WalkOuts with or without a WalkVest, your lower body will become slimmer, more toned, and more defined than ever before — and it will happen quickly. Your upper body will change too, as you are guided to use your arms, shoulders, chest, and back in the WalkOuts as well. The weight you lose will make your whole body leaner. And you'll improve your posture, protect your lower back from injury, and increase your stability by engaging your abs while you walk, which strengthens and tones your core.

Your WalkOuts will be only a part of your WorkOuts. We'll also do some additional upper, lower, and abdominal exercises to further sculpt, condition, and strengthen you. (And don't worry, you won't need extra equipment for these exercises.)

As I often tell my students, one of the best ways to improve your body's balance is to focus on strengthening the areas in which you are weak. Women, for instance, tend to neglect upper-body conditioning. The way you look in the tank top is less of a concern to me than the other areas of your life that suffer from this imbalance. Strong arms make light work of picking up (and picking up after) your children, and we need strong shoulders to carry our briefcases, not to mention the weight of the world. As men already know, strengthening your upper body makes you *feel* strong and powerful, and I want women to feel that, too.

Of course men traditionally build their upper bodies to the exclusion of aerobic exercise, which strengthens the heart and lungs. Not when they're Training for Life! This program is designed to right all our training imbalances; with the TFL programming, everyone will achieve balanced conditioning and look like it, too.

TRADE YOUR PILLS FOR A NEW PAIR OF SNEAKERS

Our bodies have astonishing regenerative powers, and it is our responsibility, as the stewards of our bodies, to give them what they need to stay healthy. Exercise is an enormous component in this ability to regenerate; I would go so far as to say that it — along with proper nutritional support — is our body's secret weapon against many of the most prevalent diseases in our culture.

In an ideal world, exercise and nutrition would eventually replace pills and injections, and I think we have the power to make it happen right now. Our body is the cure; we must give it the tools it needs to help itself. Let this knowledge influence your choices. Know that every time you choose unprocessed foods, you build the foundation for good health, and know that every time you put on your sneakers, you powerfully contribute to your body's ability to heal.

Is Walking Enough?

I've fielded the question of whether walking is sufficient hundreds of time over the years, and I completely understand the impulse to ask it. If you've finally made the decision to get into shape, you want to make sure the method you've chosen is going to be effective. Or maybe you're already walking — two or three or six times a week — but you're finding that you can't lose the weight or see any significant improvement in your level of fitness.

I'll confess, I was also skeptical that walking would be enough — in fact I was downright certain it *couldn't* be. But I now know that, done right, walking is more than enough, and I am living proof.

I was a professional long-distance athlete. I'm proud to say that I hold a world record in ultra-endurance cycling; my partner and I rode a tandem bike from California to New Jersey in just under twelve days. I rode hundreds of miles a week to train, as well as running marathons and participating in triathlons to get my body in competitive form.

When my professional athletic career ended, I still wanted to look like a pro athlete — strong, lean, and super fit — but I no longer had the time, or desire, to train like one. The answer seemed to be in shorter, more strenuous workouts, but in a few months I was feeling worn out by my routine. And when I look at old pictures now, I realize that they were making me *look* tired and old, not young and vital at all.

One day I was doing my compulsory run on the treadmill next to my friend Jim, a big football player who was known around the gym for the weighted bandoliers that he wore strapped across his chest while he walked (think Rambo). He'd been trying for months to get me to try the "progressive resistance walking" he did, but I simply didn't believe that I could get enough of a workout from walking, weights or no weights. After all, I was a fine-tuned athlete, a lean, mean, training machine, and still at the peak of my physical condition. I needed *intensity*. If a workout didn't exhaust me, physically and mentally, it couldn't possibly work.

Right?

On this day Jim wouldn't take no for an answer when I told him, "Thanks, but no thanks — walking isn't a workout." Instead he stopped his treadmill. Then he stopped MINE! Now, nobody — I don't care how big they are — messes with my workout. But before I could wrestle him to the ground, Jim had taken those bandoliers off his big shoulders, draped them over mine, and started my treadmill.

The straps were too big for me, of course, but within five minutes of walking this way, my protests died out completely. I could feel how pushing up and opposing the weight on my torso was forcing me to lengthen and strengthen my spine and improve my posture, while walking with the resistance was raising my heart rate and strengthening my muscles with every step I took. It was an incredible lower- and upper-body workout. I hated to admit it, but Jim was right.

Cut to two days later. I'm walking in my neighborhood with my own, brand-new, weighted bandoliers (think blond Rambo). As hard as it was for me to believe that plain old walking could be so effective, I was wearing the proof! My body became shapelier, stronger, and more defined in just a matter of days. The cardiovascular benefits were as powerful as they were painless, and I was really enjoying every workout again — whether I was alone or with others.

I took my commitment to this fantastic new way of getting fit to the next level when I designed WalkVest, an attractive, washable, and adjustable weight-bearing walking vest. The further away I got from being a pro athlete, the less willing I was to exercise in anything unflattering or unfashionable. (I had gotten my fair share of alarmed looks, walking through my neighborhood at six in the morning loaded with my weight bandoliers.) With WalkVest, women and men can add appropriate amounts of weight to their workouts in a comfortable and stylish way.

I have stayed committed to fitness conditioning through walking: my students and I stay spectacularly fit this way, and you can, too. Whether you're someone with a significant amount of weight to lose or just a little around the middle, whether you're a well-conditioned athlete looking to intensify and refine your training or a weekend warrior, rest assured: walking *is* enough.

Training for Life — With or Without a WalkVest

As you can probably tell, I'm a big believer in adding resistance to amp up an ordinary walking workout, but I did not write this book to sell WalkVests. You can absolutely do the Training for Life workouts — and get spectacular results — without a WalkVest, whether it's been a while since you've exercised, you have a good amount of weight to lose, or you're looking to take your training to a higher level. You don't need anything to follow the TFL program and to see fantastic changes in the way you look and feel except your own good-faith efforts.

You are the most important element in this training. The consistency and honesty with which you train, your willingness to work with me as your coach, and your own desire to succeed will change you, not your WalkVest — that can only help.

All the workouts in this book are WalkVest optional.

The coaching is why you'll feel a difference right away. I've refined and tested these WorkOuts and feel confident saying that they're the safest, most effective ones out there. And I'll happily divulge the expert training secrets I've collected from my personal and professional experience; I call them Training Tips, and you'll find them spaced throughout the WorkOuts, as if I were working out next to you. (The clever humor is just a fringe benefit.)

Once you experience how effective it is to integrate your body and mind by working on both of them together — guided by my coaching — you'll never want to go back to anything else. You'll see; it makes all the difference, to your training and to your life.

The Fundamentals: Strength, Endurance, and Recovery

The goal of Training for Life is total fitness, or as I like to say, *true* and total fitness: *true,* as in real, and *total,* as in complete. What you will learn here is entirely applicable to your life, not just your body.

Three fundamental concepts support the Training for Life conditioning practices: **strength, endurance,** and **recovery.** These concepts will act as the organizing principles of the TFL program, so that every day is either a Strength, Endurance, or Recovery Training Day, and both your WorkOuts and WorkIns will focus on some aspect of that day's fundamental principle.

These core training values provide not only a foundation for improving your *physical* self — to help you lose weight and to strengthen your muscles, bones, and cardiovascular system — but a practical and dynamic way for you to improve your inner self, as well.

I regularly have students recount stories to me about events in their lives that were improved (or made possible at all) by their training. Carol's ill child kept her awake the night before she had to make a major presentation in order to land a new account. When she woke from her scant sleep in the rocking chair by her son's bed, she felt and looked like she'd run two marathons back-to-back, and yet she had to be sharp and fresh for her presentation in just a few hours.

Calling in sick would have meant flushing six months of preparation down the drain, so Carol pulled herself together and hit the shower, repeating one of her favorite WorkIns: "My training prepares me for everything — even the unexpected." She realized that everything she'd learned from her WorkOuts and WorkIns was about to pay off. "I'm too close to the finish line to let this derail me," she thought to herself. Overcoming her exhaustion, she used everything she could muster for the final push. I'm happy to report that she nailed the presentation, and the account. Needless to say, her training had really paid off, and she felt terrific about it, even better than she would have if she'd gotten a full eight hours of sleep.

Like Carol, you'll find that working with these core training values will prove useful in *every area of your life.* Conditioning the interior "you" with compassion and consistency while you work on your exterior is how you will achieve a total transformation, not just a topical one.

Let's take a look now at how these principles apply to your body, and to your life at large.

Strength

"Lord, give me strength!"

We all need strength — and all kinds of it — at different times.

We need strength to carry life's heavy loads: the physical ones, like books, files, and children; and the mental ones, like caring for others and managing our financial responsibilities. We need strength so that we can be available to help others, whether that means moving a teenager into a dorm room or passing her tissues after her first serious breakup. We need strength to hold fast in our convictions, while still holding on to our tempers. And we need strength to take care of ourselves, so that we have the ability to recover quickly and fully from illness, discouragement, and setbacks and to ask for help when we need it.

Training for Life will give you the strength you need for all of the above — and more. You *will* strengthen your body and get rid of excess fat. But a strong body is only part of the total-fitness equation. At the same time you will empower yourself by strengthening your inner resolve.

Strength training gives you the ability to carry *any* load with ease.

To strengthen our bodies we will add resistance, and there are many ways to do that. We can increase either the weight of the load we carry or the pitch of the hill we climb. We can walk against the wind, swim against the tide, or pull something (or someone) along with us. In the process we learn to accept that resistance will condition us to better accept it in life.

If you decide to incorporate the WalkVest into your training, you'll use it with vary-ing amounts of weight to intensify your training, control the level of difficulty, and make you as formidable a force in your own unpredictable world as possible. Your strength will improve quickly, and you'll notice that you're able to do much more with greater ease. The WorkIns will empower you in a similar way. Learning to overcome difficulties makes us stronger, especially if we have effective ways of conquering them and moving beyond them, and that is what the TFL WorkIns will empower you to do.

Together the WorkOuts and WorkIns pack a powerfully beneficial punch. I have had the experience myself and seen the results of this training on others, many times over: these practices create a more powerful you. You're more present in your own life and better able to push past your comfort zone. You feel more positive, less restricted by fear, and more optimistic about what tomorrow has in store for you. You see obstacles as opportunities and resistance as a way to grow.

In this way Training for Life will give you the strength you need to live your life more powerfully — for your own benefit, and for those who count on you.

Endurance

Why do *you* think most businesses fail within twenty-four months of opening their doors? The most obvious answer is because they don't have enough money in reserve to make it through the first few years, when almost no one turns a profit.

Financial staying power is critical, of course, but money isn't the only area in which new businesses lack stamina. It takes a tremendous amount of emotional and mental re-silience to *stay the course* during a new endeavor. You must passionately believe in your idea, yourself, and your ability to make that dream come true. It takes more than money to accomplish goals. If you're going to reap the rewards of your hard work, you're going to have to ride out a lot of ups and downs along the way, and sometimes the hardest thing to do is to stay with it.

Of course the same thing is true about raising children, fixing up a house, or making a marriage work. And it's true about getting yourself into shape. You have to be able to *stay with it* in order to see the fruits of your labor. That may mean working through your fears, rising above what you consider to be sacrifice, and getting past the (in-evitable) setbacks. In order to succeed — in any of these endeavors! — you must have deep reserves, assets that you can call upon when you need sustenance, and I mean something more than a PowerBar.

You can't win if you don't make it to the finish line. And yet, as I always ask my students, how can you expect to get there if you haven't trained for it? That's why we need endurance training: life is the longest, and most important, event of all, and TFL's endurance training will give you the power to *stay on the road* and to do it with grace and ease.

There's nothing quite like *going all the way* and *giving it all you've got.*

From a strictly physical perspective, endurance training will help you burn massive amounts of excess calories, condition your cardiovascular system, and strengthen all of your body's muscles to support you through longer training sessions, as well as the long journey of life. Exercise is the fountain of youth, and endurance training, done the TFL way, will help us to combat the negative effects of aging. This training isn't just life extending, it's life *enhancing.* Life seems to get more complicated and intense with every decade — so let's get in shape for it with our training! It's not just about staying on the road, but also about staying healthy, prosperous, and vital all the way to the finish.

More important, endurance training will prepare your mind for the endurance events your life presents you with — the twelve-hour days that feel like twenty-four, those eternally unresolved personal conflicts, or just your grueling daily commute.

Endurance conditioning is also the key to *keeping* the great results you get. I know that it can be hard to keep your eye on the prize when it feels like the road is not only long but unpredictable. It's one thing to make healthy food choices when you're locked into your routine at home and another to make them on an extended business trip, especially when everyone else is pigging out! Endurance conditioning ensures that you can always live healthfully and abundantly, simply by dipping into your plentiful reserves.

When you've trained your Inner Coach with this kind of endurance conditioning, you have an internally driven support system, one that you can take with you wherever you go — and that's all you need to choose a walk over (or before) happy hour. This well-trained Inner Coach is what it means to be transformed mentally, as well as physically, and to feel as good on the inside as you do on the outside. With TFL you change much more than your waistline, and because of it, the change endures.

Recovery

Farmers periodically allow a plot of soil to lie unplanted for a season. Obviously it's more profitable for them in the short term if it's planted, but they know that the earth needs time to rejuvenate itself if it is going to be productive and abundant for years to come.

In fact, this is the key to long-term productivity and success in every arena. Baseball coaches give their star pitchers time off the mound, Fortune 500 companies send their hardworking employees on retreats, and million-dollar racehorses get rubdowns and plenty of downtime in between races. What is the lesson we can learn from these high-performance athletes and multimillion-dollar earners — not to mention Mother Nature? *The importance of recovery.* We are healthiest, and most productive, when there's enough off time incorporated into our busy schedules.

Let's face it, for most of us every day requires the concentration, stamina, and footwork of an athlete. You've got to get yourself dressed and your family fed and out the door before you put in a full day of work, then grocery shopping, dinner, other family responsibilities, and (hopefully) at least a few minutes of grown-up time before you plop into bed — it's not nothing! Then factor in time and energy for everything *else* you do, like exercising, volunteering, and maintaining a social life. Toss in a birthday party and a plumbing emergency, and you can see why you need to train as a professional athlete does.

Of course you are capable of doing all that you do; you have proven that already. But proper training can help you to do it more efficiently, less stressfully, and with more joy and ease. You'll train for the heavy lifting on your Strength Training Days and for the long haul on your Endurance Training Days. But you also have to give yourself the chance to rest, relax, and replenish your resources, as prime athletes do, and that's what we'll be doing on our Recovery Training Days.

It may seem counterintuitive, but it's true: in order for us to be at our most productive, we have to rest. That means that you must offset intervals of *intensity time* with intervals of *recovery time.* If we don't make the time to recover, we become exhausted, bored, unhealthy, resentful, and depressed. We get sick and tired of doing what we do — and we look sick and tired, too. So taking the time off — time to recover — is *not* a waste of time or a sign of laziness, as you may have been taught. Knowing what your needs are is always a sign of strength, not weakness. And when you effectively incorporate recovery time into your schedule, you feel better, you look better, and then you're ready for anything.

Recovery is essential to making the most of your time and your abilities.

Training for Life, as we said just a minute ago, is about total fitness, and a huge part of total fitness is learning to take good care of yourself. *There is no greater act of self-care than making sure you have enough time to rest.* Overtraining is like overspending (a concept you're probably familiar with) — it leaves you exhausted from always trying to catch up. Athletes know how to rest their bodies and their minds effectively so that they're ready to rise to any challenge at any time; in Training for Life we go a step further, because as athletes in training for *life,* you never know when the next challenge will present itself. That's why we treat the act of recovery with the same respect and importance that we do every other part of our training.

You'll note that a Recovery Training Day isn't necessarily a day of complete rest; instead it's a very low-intensity training day. Why not just take the day off? Because the idea here is to train you *for life,* and unless you have a much better situation than I do, there aren't many days of doing absolutely nothing in life. Weekends might be more relaxing than weekdays, but when was the last time you had a Saturday with absolutely no responsibilities — no soccer games, no dogs to groom, no storm drains to clean, no dry cleaning to drop off? No e-mails to answer, no phone calls to return, no work to catch up on, no bills to pay? I thought so. Because real days of no responsibilities are few and far between in your life, so will they be in our training, but that doesn't mean you can't rest.

In fact most of us regularly pass by opportunities to recover because we aren't trained to recognize them. But taking advantage of these unseen respites would make your work, and your day, much easier and more enjoyable. I can't give you a week on a deserted beach in Tahiti, but I can show you how to identify, and make the most of, these opportunities when they occur.

Everyone's recovery is personal. For you it might be taking a break in the middle of a crazy afternoon to walk around the block or to close your door for five minutes so you can shut your eyes or read a magazine. Sometimes it means making time for a nap, a vacation, or just a bath at the end of the day. No matter what it is, it must be a regular part of your schedule. And as you progress, you'll begin to realize how much recovery time you need, based on your own personality and the intensity of your lifestyle.

Don't wait until it's too late. That's when you start to make the choices that can sabotage your healthy lifestyle and well-being, starting a negative spiral that gets harder and harder to break. Burning out leads to choices like eating lots of sugary foods to fuel you as you work late — or courting injury by going to the gym to burn off those extra calories, even when you feel tired or weak. Or giving up exercise altogether because you're mentally and physically exhausted, and working out feels like the straw that's going to break the camel's back. Recovery isn't effective if you wait until you're completely toasted to take a rest; that's not recovery, it's hitting bottom. You don't have to let it go that far.

I will show you how to use the recovery times that present themselves to you over the course of your day. As a result you will find that you have more energy, and reserve energy when you need it. You will find that there is *always* time to recover, not necessarily when you *want* it, but when you *need* it.

So strength, endurance, and recovery are the three central concepts we'll be working with in *Training for Life,* and every day, both your WorkOut and WorkIn will be focused on a specific facet of one of them. I hope that you'll reflect upon how these fundamentals apply, not just to your workouts and body, but to every aspect of your life.

Total Fitness: It's Not About the Numbers

Before you begin this fourteen-day program, I want you to get on the scale and weigh in, and then I want you to put your scale away — at least until the end of the fourteen days.

In general we're way too focused on what I call "the numbers." My students ask me, "How much will I lose in the first week?" (Answer: nobody can answer that question with any certainty.) "How many calories will I burn doing each WorkOut?" (Another question with too many variables to accurately answer.) Ditto for "What's my body fat percentage, and what *should* it be?"

All these numbers are just distractions.

What exactly do all these numbers mean to you anyway? If you knew what the answers to those questions were, would you be more easily able to reach your goals and maintain your results? I think the opposite is true. When you create expectation (the way you do when you set a goal weight — "128 or bust!") you create a predisposition to failure — the way you have, over and over again, on the programs you've tried in the past.

I realize that asking you to set aside these numbers may be like asking you to give up breathing. For most of us these numbers are integral to the way we think about fitness. We've been long conditioned to believe that these numbers hold some magic importance; if we only knew the right ones, they'd give us the ticket out of the situation we find ourselves in. So we use calipers to determine our body-fat content, we weigh ourselves at different times during the day, and we calculate how many fat grams we've just eaten. Obsessing about these numbers has become our new national pastime; I think it's bigger than baseball!

Unfortunately this preoccupation is also one that completely opposes long-term weight loss, good health, and total fitness. These numbers are just a marketing tool used by the diet and weight-loss industry — a multibillion-dollar phenomenon that we have created simply by agreeing to get (and stay) on the diet-go-round. We start a diet, fail at it (of course — because we can't reach or maintain those magic numbers), abandon our efforts, feel guilty, start another diet, fail, and so it goes. Every year the diet and weight-loss industry expands — selling more and more products and programs to Americans to help them lose weight — while American men, women, and children continue to expand, too, getting heavier and unhealthier each year. It's a system that profits no one except the people selling the diets.

It seems tragic to me that we've made the marketers of diet and weight-loss products the keepers of our bodies. We have been primed to do it by our conditioning: weren't we all taught at a young age to listen to "the experts"? We learned that teachers and doctors are always right, and that if it's on TV, it must be true. So we buy what they tell us to buy, and when it fails after a couple of months, we buy something else. We put our trust and our hopes in a fantasy: "thinner thighs in ten days!" "a product that will melt away fat, or your money back!" And in so doing, we support an industry that doesn't respect, support, or benefit us in any way.

A better way exists, but it requires your consent to change.

The nineteenth-century philosopher and economist J. S. Mill wrote, "No great improvements in the lot of mankind are possible, until a great change takes place in the fundamental constitution of their modes of thought." I believe that we need to engineer a revolution in the way we think about our bodies and in the very way that we define fitness and health.

The goal of Training for Life is total fitness, and it encompasses much, much more than "the numbers." You might be thinking that nothing is more important to you than losing the weight — and fast! But what about losing the weight *and keeping it off*? How about improving your sense of self-respect and your self-esteem? What about happiness? What would you say to the possibility of a total mental and physical transformation?

That's why Training for Life isn't solely a weight-loss program.

**Weight loss certainly is a component of fitness,
but it is not the *definition* of fitness.**

And TFL isn't a diet either, although it does have a diet component to it. This program doesn't put how much weight you can lose in a short period of time ahead of what I consider to be *true* fitness concerns, like long-term weight loss, muscle and bone strength, cardiovascular endurance, and your total well-being. And the funny thing is that doing it right isn't harder and doesn't take any longer — it's simply more effective.

The conditioning you'll do as part of Training for Life is designed to help you to think differently about fitness. And this conditioning will ensure that the total fitness you achieve *lasts*. I don't believe that any change that happens to your body (including weight loss) because of dieting and exercising can last or truly benefit you unless it is done with mental conditioning as well.

Let's get one thing straight: I'm not offering you a magic formula, because there isn't one. But I can show you how to get in touch with and use qualities that already exist within you, qualities that will *guarantee* your long-term success. You will not be spending your time in this program trying to hit a specific number — not a goal weight, not a certain number of calories a day, and not a deadline to lose a certain number of pounds. As you'll see in the next chapter, the only scale that you'll need to do Training for Life is called Your Effort Scale, and it's a measurement of your own efforts.

Soon "goal weight" will no longer be the most important phrase in your fitness vocabulary. Your goals will shift from quick weight loss to long-term weight loss; from "how many inches can I lose?" to "how much freedom can I gain?" You'll go from watching the numbers on the scale to seeing your strength, happiness, and youthfulness increase. Success is a state of mind, as well as a new state of body. It's not just how you look that changes your life, but how you feel, and how you *are*. When you get off the diet-go-round, you're free to dedicate yourself to living a life that is joyful, comfortable, useful, prosperous, and healthy rather than one that is entirely consumed with the newest way to drop weight.

And all you have to do to achieve total fitness is to follow along with Training for Life. Little by little, step by step, and day by day, you'll find that everything falls into place. "But how will I know it's working?" you're wondering. All I can say is that you'll know. So begin to embrace letting go of the concept of a "goal weight," and we'll begin to think instead about your goals for your life, not just your body. Isn't that the true definition of success?

My friend Bari joined me for dinner the other day. "You look terrific," I told her —
and she did! She smiled and said,

> You know, my belly could be flatter, and I could do with a little less wiggle in my upper
> arms, but I feel damn good — better at forty-nine than I did at thirty-nine, for sure. I feel
> great, I look good in my clothes, and I'm healthier than I've ever been — and it's no chore
> to maintain. I eat healthy, whole foods (most of the time, anyway), I work out five times a
> week, and I still have plenty of time and energy for work and my family. That's all I need
> to remember when I see someone in a magazine who makes me feel like I should be
> thinner.

Bari hasn't been on a scale in two years, but she knows she's achieved her goal, and I can
help you get there, too. Let me help you remove the distraction of those numbers so
you can concentrate on what's really important: *the way you feel.* That is the true measure of your progress. You need to do your WorkOuts so that you *look* better and your
WorkIns so that you *feel* better, and if you let go of distractions like "the numbers," you
will *experience* the changes and know for sure that you're improving. If you focus on
your actions rather than results, you really will lose weight, and you'll get fit — totally
fit — for good.

CHAPTER 6

Setup for Success: The Basics

T raining for Life doesn't require you to spend a great deal of time and money in preparation, but you'll need to be familiar with some fundamental concepts and training tools before we start. In this chapter I'll walk you through what you need and what you need to know.

What You'll Need

A Positive Attitude

> *"Ability is what you're capable of doing. Motivation determines what you do. Attitude determines how well you do it."*
>
> —LOU HOLTZ

The first thing you'll need is a positive attitude. As part of your training, I'm asking you to usher in a whole new way of thinking, and that new way of thinking starts here. When you're Training for Life, a positive attitude doesn't mean "I know I can lose twenty-five pounds by the reunion" or "I'll work really hard for two weeks and get rid of my spare tire." That's not a positive attitude; it's unrealistic expectation and a sure setup for failure — just the way you've set yourself up for failure in the past.

You'll be doing something different this time, and that difference will mean letting go of all of your old, self-defeating notions — like the idea that you can predict or control your results. You can't determine how quickly the weight will leave you, only how much effort you are willing to give toward improved fitness every day.

Training for Life is a process. The more diligently and consistently you train, the more likely it is that your body will change quickly. Letting go of your results doesn't mean that we're not working conscientiously toward a sleek physique and slender, sexy body. Your body will get better, substantially better — and so will your life. But you cannot decide what will happen to your body, or when, before we even begin. You have to let go of those expectations.

When you do, you eliminate some of the most devious pitfalls that may have snared you in the past. No magic will give you the body you want. You must agree to work hand in hand with me, delivering your purest efforts, so that together we can condition and improve you, body and mind.

More than anything, a positive attitude means accepting that you truly *are* capable of attaining your weight, health, and fitness goals, as well as sustaining them permanently — and it won't be hard because, for the first time, you'll have the tools you need to make it happen. While the WorkOuts are designed to rapidly improve the way your body looks and feels, the WorkIns that you will do are designed to change your mind, improve your self-esteem, and give you a new outlook — one that makes it easy for you to be consistent and dedicated to this new way of living.

That's the setup for success.

A NEW AGE OF AWARENESS: LISTENING TO YOUR BODY

I'm always struck by how little attention we pay to our bodies; it seems that we know very little about how to protect, care for, and improve them compassionately. In my opinion, this stems from a fundamental lack of awareness.

Let me give you an example from my own life. A couple of years ago, I suffered a lower-back injury. Was it the result of overtraining or an accident on the road? No. It was the result of cumulative minor trauma over time — incurred *by the way I get in and out of my car.* I'd been throwing myself behind the wheel of my car (you know what I'm talking about) two, four, sometimes ten times a day since I got my license. It took an injury for me to realize (the way I finally realized that smoking wasn't good for me, drinking wasn't good for me, overeating wasn't good for me, and even that *running* wasn't good for me) that I had been ignoring the very clear signs my body had been sending me — in this case a tweak in my lower back every time I got behind the wheel.

As our bodies age they become more fragile and sensitive. We can take a significant step toward preserving our youthfulness simply by becoming more sensitive to our body's needs and restrictions. Unfortunately I now have a painful "red flag" in my lower back that reminds me, when I'm doing too much or not paying enough attention, to treat my body compassionately. That little reminder makes me much more cautious about the way I get into my car — and that's just the beginning. I pay attention to how I sit at my desk, in a movie theater, or in my favorite reading chair. I walk carefully in heels (and even in my workout shoes), cautious about where and how I step. I wear supportive fitness shoes, even just to walk the dogs. Perhaps most important, I try to recognize when my body is tired, whether I'm swinging a golf club or working in my office, so that I can prevent injury and illness rather than spending weeks sidelined because of my own behavior.

Training for Life will automatically raise your physical awareness by virtue of the exercises you will be doing, while the WorkIns will improve your mental and emotional awareness as well. Hopefully you will use this newfound awareness to learn how to attend more healthfully to your physical self. Note the spots that feel vulnerable and the activities that strain them *before* they become injuries, and take steps to protect your body and your new way of life. With this new awareness you won't have to succumb to the aches and pains of age — at least not those that you can prevent.

Now, on to the basics.

Clothes

I don't care what clothes you work out in, as long as they're comfortable, breathable, and appropriate for the climate you're in. You're going to be working out often, so whether you splurge on designer tracksuits or opt for your son's old T-shirts, make sure you have enough items so that you'll have clean, fresh clothes every day.

Shoes

Sneaker technology is a big business, and the selection can be a little overwhelming. To keep it simple I recommend that my students look for shoes designed for either walking or long-distance running. Both types will have ample support and provide comfort over the long haul.

I personally prefer a long-distance running shoe. Although running and walking are very different activities, a lot of money and engineering have gone into creating products that cushion the joints and muscles of people who run long and short distances on every surface you can imagine. I want that expensive technology protecting my joints and muscles and those of my students. As fitness walking rises in popularity, shoe companies are spending more energy and greater resources on developing products that target the particular needs of walkers, so try on both types and see what feels most comfortable to you.

The first exercise for your Inner Coach will be making sure you get the shoes that are best for your feet. Everyone's feet are different; don't be surprised if even a top-of-the-line shoe feels uncomfortable. How will you know you've found the right pair? First and foremost, your shoes should be comfortable *right off the bat*. They should feel good in the store; I can tell you from experience that a shoe that isn't comfortable as soon as you slip your foot into it isn't going to be any more comfortable after an hour's workout. If there's any question in your mind about whether you've found the right pair, keep shopping.

You shouldn't wear your brand-new shoes for the first time during a training session. Wear them around the house and to the store a couple of times to break them in a little bit. Once you've broken them in, wear them only for training.

You'll want to replace your shoes every three to six months if you're walking four to six days a week. Keep an eye on the soles and note how quickly they wear down. And if your heels or knees or shins get sore after walking pain free for a couple of months, that may be a sign that your shoes are no longer providing the support that you need from them. Don't wait until you get injured! Use the body awareness you'll gain from doing Training for Life to recognize the signs, and replace your shoes so you don't have to hang them up while you're recuperating.

What You Need to Know

Walking Basics

When you're walking for fitness, the way your foot strikes the ground is important if you want to get the best workout possible and avoid injury. It's not realistic to expect you to change your stride completely at this stage in your life, but you can bring a heightened sense of awareness to certain aspects of the way you walk.

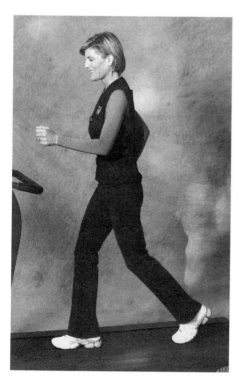

When your foot strikes the ground, roll over your heel instead of hitting the ground with it. Then push off from the ball of your foot. Walking this way will protect you from unnecessary impact. It will also give you greater momentum and the ability to easily increase your pace while keeping your natural stride intact.

Your posture while you walk is also very important. Keep your chin level with the ground or tilted down ever so slightly. Walk tall, as if there were a string attached to the top of your head, and drop your shoulders so that you look naturally poised. Correcting your posture this way not only improves the way you look but also elongates and opens your spine, creating space for energy to flow efficiently through your body. Believe it or not, this improved flow of energy will fuel and sustain you, allowing you to go beyond your previous limits. By training efficiently, you can *get* more without *doing* more.

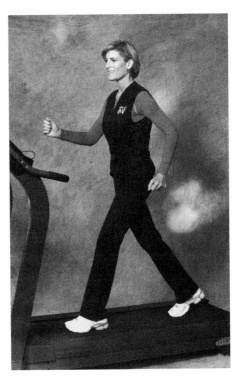

Check with your posture periodically. Most of all, don't overthink your stride: the goal is to move as fluidly and naturally as you can. The more you do it, the more natural it will become.

Note to Your Inner Coach

Posture isn't just physical; you have a mental and emotional posture as well. So when you scan your body to make sure that your chest is open and your shoulders are back and that your abs are engaged, or pulled in, check in with your mind as well. Is your positive attitude open and engaged as well? Regularly scanning *all* of these postures will ensure that you have a maximally beneficial training session each day.

WalkVest Basics

The WalkVest is optional, which means that every WalkOut in this book can be done very effectively without it.

As you get fitter, however, you may decide that you want to make your WorkOuts more powerful without increasing the amount of time you spend on them. Safely adding resistance to your WorkOuts allows you to burn more fat and calories, builds cardiovascular strength and bone density, and helps to sculpt and tone your body. So using a WalkVest gives you the opportunity to *get* more without *doing* more. It makes your WorkOuts — or just a trip to the grocery store — more powerful and effective.

What Is the WalkVest?

The WalkVest is a lightweight cotton vest, with pockets located around your torso. You load these pockets with half-pound weight bars, distributing them evenly among the front and back and right and left sides.

Tighten the belts around your waist and chest until your WalkVest fits snugly and securely against your body. The core support belt, located at your waistline, is especially important. Keeping it snugly fastened will keep the weights from bouncing against your body and remind you to engage your abdominal muscles. This will condition those muscles as well as support your lower back and will improve your posture at the same time. To tighten, fasten the plastic buckle and then hold it tightly with one hand while you pull the belt strap end with the other.

How Much Weight Should I Use?

For most people, the four pounds that come in the basic WalkVest package is an appropriate amount of weight to use at the beginning. People who are very new to exercise, extremely small (under a hundred pounds), or recovering from an injury should begin with two pounds (four bars).

If you're very fit, four pounds may not feel like enough. I trust you (and your inner coach) to know when you need a greater challenge; there's no better indication that you need to add weight than feeling like you're not sufficiently "worked out" after a WalkOut, even though you have diligently followed my training instructions. When that happens you can purchase more weight (your WalkVest holds up to sixteen pounds).

Always add weight gradually (in two-pound increments), so your body can safely adjust. If you discover that you feel extremely fatigued or overly sore after a WalkOut, you should probably reduce the amount of weight in your WalkVest by two pounds for a little while.

In the eight years since I developed the WalkVest, I've been asked the following question hundreds of times, so if you don't mind, I'm going to anticipate and answer it here:

Question: I'm overweight — why isn't the excess weight I'm already carrying making me fit?

Answer: Gaining weight happens slowly over time. As you gain, your body adapts; it programs itself to know how much energy it will need to expend to carry you through your day.

The weight you add when you put on a WalkVest is unfamiliar to your body, *different* from the body weight you carry around all day, every day. So your body responds to *that* added weight uniquely, creating what athletes call a "training effect." Adding weight with a WalkVest instantly demands that your body exert more energy to sustain the weight and move you around. Your body has to work harder, so you burn more calories, and the extra work that your muscles and bones have to do to support the extra weight has an intensified strengthening and toning effect on them.

Strengthening, Toning, and Stretching Basics

Every workout will end with a session that combines some strengthening, toning, and/or stretching exercises.

Toning

As you do your toning and strengthening exercises, I'd like you to stay aware and in control. Take your time with each movement; when you rush, you only cheat yourself out of an effective WorkOut and expose yourself to greater injury potential. Stay in touch with your body! Deliver your best efforts, and you'll reap the rewards.

OUCH — IT HURTS!

Over the course of the next fourteen days, you may be feeling muscles you didn't even know you had. While some muscle soreness is to be expected, it's always most intense when you begin exercising after some time away.

You may be a little uncomfortable, but if you can see this soreness as a positive sign — a signal from your body that it's going through some very powerful changes — you can embrace it.

In the meantime here's what everyone should do to safely condition and recover your muscles:

Take hot baths: Soreness was a real problem for me when I was training to ride my bike across the country; I dealt with it (and, I believe, escaped sustained injury) because of this age-old trick: fill a bathtub to hip level, with just enough water to cover your legs and two cups of Epsom salts — and make it as hot as you can take it! Sit in there for five minutes minimum (twenty minutes is best — bring a magazine). Keeping the water level low will help you tolerate the heat, and soaking in all that heat will help the muscles in your lower body to loosen and release. If it's your upper body that's sore, you'll have to fill it all the way up; stay hydrated while soaking, and get out immediately if you feel yourself getting dizzy or light-headed.

Stay warm: Cold muscles are tight muscles, which makes them easier to injure, and they're never more vulnerable than when transitioning from hot to cold, so keep yourself warm! Make sure you have warm clothing to keep the heat in after you've worked out, even if you're just going to your car. And when exiting your hot bath, dry off and wrap up well.

Move! If your muscles are sore, sit on the floor and do a little stretching while you watch TV or go for an extra-gentle, restorative walk with your kids or the dog. Keep it easy and smooth — even ten minutes will help by increasing the blood flow to the muscle groups that hurt.

Training for Life is intense, but it is compassionate. You may be sore, but your WorkOuts shouldn't leave you incapacitated; if they do, it's a sign to your Inner Coach that you need to back off and do a little less. I love the way it feels to "feel" my body, and you will, too. I love to feel the strength in my legs with every step, the power in my upper body as I go about my daily activities, and the security of my core. No matter what your weight, age, or physical condition is right now, this is entirely within your reach — and you'll experience what I'm talking about in the next fourteen days.

Stretching

No one — myself included — stretches enough. Stretching helps improve posture, balance, strength, and endurance. It makes you less likely to injure yourself. Gentle, compassionate, and consistent stretching will enhance muscle recovery and ease soreness. Furthermore, research has indicated that stretching can make your muscles react more effectively to resistance training; in other words, stretching is another way you can get more by training more efficiently. Best of all, it feels great!

Probably the biggest myth about stretching is that you should do it *before* you work out. **WRONG. Never stretch before your muscles are warmed up.** Your muscles are more flexible and less likely to tear when they're warm. Don't worry: you will be more than adequately prepared for every WorkOut session; every WalkOut begins with a segment of gentle walking, which gives your muscles the opportunity to warm up before the real work begins and gives you the chance to check in and see how your body feels. Feel free to experiment with your range of motion during these segments: roll your shoulders and swing your arms gently across your body; walk with your knees lifted high or lift your heels back toward your rear end. In fact I love to get off the treadmill and do a short stretching session after my warm-up and before my WalkOut, but if you don't have the time (as I usually don't), reserve the real stretching for after your WorkOut, when you'll get the most out of it.

When you stretch:

- Hold every stretch for a minimum of ten seconds.
- Stretching is all about walking the fine line between "enough" and "too much" — never force a stretch. Use the awareness you're honing, and stay in tune with your body; it *should* feel like a stretch, but it shouldn't hurt.

A NEW AGE OF AWARENESS: MIND TO YOUR MUSCLES

I often encourage my students to "bring their mind to their muscles" when they stretch.

All I'm really asking for is the added awareness that comes when you bring your concentration to the specific muscle group the stretch is designed to target. Like a magnifying glass catching the rays of the sun, your mind can act as a powerful focusing and intensifying device, dramatically increasing the effectiveness of the stretch.

- *Don't* bounce.
- *Don't* worry about how far you can go; some people are very flexible, and some people aren't (and most people are more flexible in some areas of their bodies than in others). Everyone benefits from the effort, no matter what it looks like, and it will look (and feel) significantly better by the end of these fourteen days; I guarantee it!
- *Don't* be concerned if you go farther on one side than you can on the other; that's perfectly normal. Simply do what you can and note the difference.
- *Don't* forget to breathe! Try this: inhale, and as you let the breath out through your nose, go a little farther into the stretch.

Where to Work Out

One of the best things about walking is that you can do it anywhere: you can hike in the hills; hit the neighborhood pavement; go to a gym, a park, or a school track; or do laps around the mall.

I prefer that you do your TFL WalkOuts on a treadmill for one reason: you have more control. You won't encounter rain, bad drivers, or unknown terrain, which means that you'll be able to have a seamless, safe, and effective training session every time (but if you do not have access to a treadmill, that's okay; I'll discuss this later). You'll still have plenty of distractions to work through on a treadmill — like televisions, determined conversationalists posing as workout enthusiasts, and (my favorite) exhibitionists in inappropriate workout attire — but you'll learn to keep your focus as part of your training.

Treadmills come with a variety of bells and whistles — I recommend that you use only the timing, speed, and elevation functions. Trust your body: treadmills may be calibrated differently so that three miles per hour may feel much faster on one than another. Simply use the up and down keys to increase and decrease your pace and incline; it's not about how fast you're going, anyway.

Although I do prefer that you walk on a treadmill, it's certainly not essential. The best thing about walking is that lack of access isn't ever an excuse — you can always walk outdoors, no matter where you are. If you take your WorkOuts outside, try to choose a route you know and one where you can do your training without interruption. If you walk where there are cars, wear clothing that's easy to see from a distance (the

WalkVest has reflective logos on front and back). And if you are walking with someone else, make sure that they're also Training for Life — or at least not interfering with your training.

For the first fourteen days, I'm going to ask you to leave your strollers and dogs at home so you can follow my training as it is written (or on CD). In these early days please devote your full concentration to getting the most from your training efforts.

Your Effort Scale (YES)

In order to guide you through different levels of intensity in your WorkOuts, we need an accurate way to measure intensity. And it must be personalized, since each of us is different, and we'll all be training together. No matter what your age, size, experience, or level of fitness, Training for Life is right for you. Novices can train for life, and so can experienced athletes; twenty-somethings can do it, and so can their grandparents.

That's why, as you read the instructions for your WorkOuts, you'll see something unique to TFL. Instead of telling you what speed your treadmill should be at, or how fast your heart should be beating, I use a measurement called YES. It stands for *Your Effort Scale,* and it is the most precise instrument I know of to make sure that you're taking responsibility and putting *into* your WorkOuts what you hope to get *out.* As with everything in life, what you give is what you get. You control the single greatest determining factor in your results: *the effort that you bring* to every WorkOut and WorkIn.

That's the good news: your potent and committed efforts will always bring you dramatic results. But it's also the bad news: if your effort is meek, your results will be, too. YES is a measure of *your effort* — that's it. It puts the responsibility of evaluating, increasing, and decreasing your effort squarely on YOU. I can't tell you what your heart rate should be at, and I can't tell you how many miles per hour you should be going on the treadmill (not to mention that every machine is different). What I *can* tell you — and will, at varying points during your WorkOuts — is how much *effort* you need to give to get the best overall results. You'll determine how much intensity you need to deliver in order to match the effort I'm asking you for by increasing the speed (and incline if you are on a treadmill) at which you walk.

So what you have to do is manage your walking speed and the incline that you walk at to find the level of activity that makes you feel YES as I have described it. The beauty of

	YES	WHAT IT FEELS LIKE
EASY ZONE	1	Very easy, requiring very little effort. The speed at which you'd window-shop or stroll through the park. Your breathing feels normal.
	2	Gentle, mild effort; your body still feels comfortable, although your breathing is slightly more noticeable than at YES 1.
	3	Gentle effort. Your breathing is still at a comfortable level, but a little deeper than YES 2, and you should feel your muscles beginning to get warm.
MODERATE ZONE	4	Gently engaged. You're walking with a purpose, as if to a meeting.
	5	Engaged. You're walking as if you're late to that meeting. Your body is very warm.
	6	Completely engaged; you feel like you're engaged in exercise! Your breathing is deep, although you can probably carry on a (slightly winded) conversation with the person on the treadmill next to you.
POWER ZONE	7	Deeply engaged. You'd be hard-pressed to answer a question with more than a word or two, and you can feel that your heart rate is elevated. Your muscles are purposefully engaged, and you can feel each muscle group doing its work.
	8	Seriously engaged. This should feel close to the upper limits of what you can do. Speaking would be very difficult, if not impossible.
	9	Extremely engaged. This is your maximum and can't be maintained for very long. Your breathing is stressed and will be difficult to catch, but we won't be here for long, and this is very effective fat-burning and heart-strengthening work.
	10	Flat-out effort, as if you were fleeing from danger. If you were asked to expend this level of effort, you likely never could. World-class athletes may reach this level in their racing after much training, but you and I will probably never get here. If you did, it would probably take more recovery than we are scheduled to do, and that is not our best use of time and resources. But by participating in TFL, you will soon be better prepared to execute an all-out effort if you are ever required to do so.

this system is that it allows me to deliver individualized, personalized coaching to everyone, no matter your age, weight, level of fitness, or state of health. YES is relative to YOU. Because your level of effort is the guidepost, your level of intensity will always be perfectly calibrated to you.

Let me show you what I mean. Carl is a sixty-six-year-old ex-smoker, more than a hundred pounds overweight, and recuperating from his second heart attack; Violet is a fit thirty-three-year-old who has run a marathon every year since her twentieth birthday. When Carl is delivering a YES of 6 (a fairly engaged pace), it will probably look substantially different — slower — than the pace of Violet's 6, but that is exactly how it is supposed to be.

As long as the effort you expend (YES) matches what I have asked you for, you'll be getting the WorkOut you need for the best results possible.

And as Carl begins to shed his excess weight and increase his cardiovascular strength, *his own* YES 6 will look very different than it does today.

The YES scale goes from 1 to 10. As you get more experienced, you'll get a feel for what YES 6 should feel like, but you may want to bookmark the page so that you can easily return to it for reference in the beginning.

YES puts YOU in the driver's seat. You determine your effort expenditure and, therefore, the results. Training for Life gives you everything you need to get fit — exceptionally fit — and stay that way. But your level of improvement, the amount of weight loss, and the time it takes for you to realize your goals is dependent on your level of attention and commitment and on a truly praiseworthy effort.

Don't sell yourself short, and don't underestimate my aspirations for you. To reach your potential you must be the honor-bound monitor of your efforts. In the end, and always, we are the wisest guardians of our own health. With my guidance and your best efforts, we will have all we need to create the results you want.

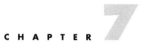

A Clean Diet

With exercise you can radically change your body and improve your health. But there is another important factor in the health-and-fitness equation: food.

What you eat is a significant — I might even say enormous — factor in how you look and feel. By extension it determines how actively and joyfully you participate in your life. But the role food plays in our lives is more complicated than it appears on the surface, which is why it's so often a tricky part of the weight-loss equation.

How Did We Get Here?

Food is a source of energy, and it can also be a source of pleasure. But many of us eat past the point of pleasure and eat much more than we need to live. We eat for reasons that have nothing to do with survival — or physical survival, anyway. We do use food for "emotional survival": as reward and punishment and to suppress anger, resentment, fear, sadness, and sometimes even the discomfort that joy and success can bring.

Traditional diets fail to take our multidimensional, complex relationship with food into account — no wonder they fail! In my opinion most of them should come with a cautionary sticker like the ones you find on cigarette packs: "Warning: This diet may change your body — but not for long."

Some diets are too restrictive or confusing to follow in real life, and some are downright unhealthy, but the real problem is that *all* of them foster what I call the "on" and "off" mentality: the idea that you're either "on" a diet or "off" it, which gives way to a whole cycle of damaging feelings and behaviors — like guilt, self-hatred, and out-of-control overeating.

Don't be surprised if it sounds familiar: this cycle of restriction and indulgence has been the backbone of the traditional American diet of the twenty-first century, and the on/off formula is now deeply etched into our minds. We have subscribed to the process, adopted the mind-set, and agreed (time after time!) to get on board the diet-go-round. We're heavier and sicker than we've ever been and desperate for a way out, so we believe them when they say that *this* new diet will change us fast and for the better. No wonder the diet and weight-loss industry is thriving! But they're the only ones who are.

Getting Off the Diet-Go-Round

You can — and must — break free of this cycle. We have traded common sense for promises of *thinner faster* for far too long; it's time to put a stop to our collusion with the fraud. And by buying this book, you have asked for my help. It's not a responsibility I take lightly: I'm calling for nothing less than a revolution.

Training for Life isn't just about losing weight; it's about changing your lifestyle in order to change your body and improve your life forever. Maybe you feel like you've heard that line before: keep listening. Getting there will take a radical shift away from the traditional on/off dieting mind-set. In order to succeed, you must change your beliefs, about weight loss and about you. In the next fourteen days, I will show you how, and I will personally help you do it.

> **Understanding yourself is just as important as understanding which food choices are healthiest; I'll help you with both.**

I intend to provide you with a great deal more than just a diet. By the time these fourteen days are up, you will understand why you continue to overeat, even though you say that you desperately want to lose weight.

The First Fourteen Days

At the beginning my recommendations *will* look like a diet; in fact, following the dietary specifications that I provide for you will be very important. There's plenty of reconditioning that must take place, and it must come from a source other than your mind, the current source of all your unhealthy thoughts and behaviors! In a sense it will be just like "doing" a diet, but the goal isn't just to get you back into your skinny jeans — it's to make sure that your skinny jeans become your *always* jeans, by teaching you a whole new way of thinking about yourself and your food.

For the first fourteen days, you will have to rely on me and your self-discipline. Now I *don't* expect you to rely on either one of those things for very long: that way of life is too joyless to sustain, and it's not the kind of life I'm training you for. But for these first two weeks, you will have to dig deep, to access a level of commitment and perseverance that you may not have used in quite a while; but don't worry, it *is* available to everyone. I guarantee it.

As time goes on, the training that you'll be given will enable you to recognize and change your patterns of unhealthy eating — with or without me — so that you're more in control of your food choices and your life. Practice and repetition can alter any habit, including overeating. You are going to clean up your diet on the outside and change your feelings about it on the inside.

A NEW AGE OF AWARENESS: CHOOSING EVERY BITE

"OK," you think as you flip through the food plans in this book, "I can do that for fourteen days. But I'm worried about what will happen to me after that."

Given the average American's history on the diet-go-round, that's a perfectly legitimate concern. I don't doubt that you have the self-discipline to get you through the first fourteen days, but I don't want you to have to rely on self-discipline forever — mostly because it won't work. When you train for life, you don't have to white-knuckle your food choices or your life. Instead you'll gain awareness, the most important tool in the Training for Life program.

**The way to easily sustain a healthier diet
is by increasing your *awareness*.**

Nothing is more important in life than the ability to make conscious, well-informed choices, and that takes awareness. Having awareness doesn't mean that you'll never eat a chocolate-chip cookie again; it does mean, though, that you'll never do it without realizing it or without wanting to. If you're going to have a cookie, I want you to choose it, not eat it unconsciously and hate yourself afterward.

This awareness will develop naturally, through the training that we do together during this program. I will set out clear food choices and boundaries for you to follow. This, accompanied by the healthy mind-body conditioning practices you'll be doing over the next fourteen days, will give you a powerful new way of deciding what you will eat and how you will eat it. We will focus on personal responsibility and accountability in every area of your life — including the dinner table and the grocery store. With some practice, your thoughts (and behaviors) can change for good.

The more aware you are, the easier it is to make healthy choices. Your body will change, and you will look better; but more important, you will become a person who makes healthier choices consistently and loves the way it feels.

A Clean Diet

I call the diet I recommend to my students (and the one I follow myself) a "clean" diet. A clean diet is one that has *less* refined foods (like white flour, refined sugar, fried foods, and prepackaged bars and meal replacements) and *more* whole and unprocessed foods, like vegetables, whole grains, and lean meats. There's *less* alcohol, caffeine, and artificial sweeteners and *more* water. There will be no grazing, no filling up on soda, and no gum chewing. There will be *no more* eating in bed, in your car, late at night, or unconsciously. And there will be *no* "blowing it" and starting over.

A clean diet is as flexible as you want it to be, especially as you get more confident about the choices you make. It uses foods that are widely available everywhere; you'll be able to follow my recommendations whether you're at a friend's house, in a restaurant, on vacation, or stuck in the airport. When you train for life, there are no rules, only guidelines; after all, my goal is to help you find practical ways to eat the most responsible, healthy, and enjoyable diet possible, for the rest of your life.

Training for Life Clean Diet Guidelines

- Eat moderately sized meals. That means four to six ounces (a fist-size serving) of protein, one-third to two-thirds of a cup of cooked whole grains, and one to two cups of cooked vegetables. Be even more generous with green vegetables.
- Eat three meals a day, with two optional snacks/mini meals.
- Eat as many different varieties and colors of vegetables and fruits as you can every day.
- When you can, buy fresh vegetables and fruits over frozen, and frozen over canned.
- Buy organic vegetables and fruits whenever possible, and choose antibiotic- and hormone-free meats.

EATING WITH AWARENESS

Over the last few years, I have become more educated about compassionate farming practices. I feel better, physically and emotionally, when I know that my food was produced with respect for its source — whether that source is an animal or the Earth herself.

I limit my family's exposure to pesticides by buying organic fruits and vegetables, and I recommend that you seek out hormone- and antibiotic-free meat. The phrases "free-range," "free-grazing," and "grass-fed" or "pasture-fed" are all indications that the animal was raised in a more natural environment.

These choices are a little more expensive, but worth it.

- Choose proteins that are high in vitamins and rich in important nutrients. I recommend fish like salmon, fresh or canned tuna, halibut, sole, and other white fish; soy products like tofu, tempeh, and soy burgers; as well as chicken and turkey.
- Vegetables may be steamed or grilled; the longer they cook, the more nutrients they lose.
- When I call for soup, homemade is best, but canned or frozen versions (such as those made by Hain or Progresso) can be substituted, as long as they have no

sugar, no dairy, and not more than three grams of fat per serving. Commercial versions can be very high in sodium; if you're watching your sodium intake, make sure to choose a low-sodium or sodium-free product.

- Salad dressing, if not homemade, should be all natural, with no sugar and no artificial sweeteners. Splurge on a dressing you really love and don't worry about the fat; treat it like a delicacy and use it sparingly. Different vinegars (balsamic, red wine, sherry, or rice) or lemon juice can also be used to add flavor to salads or cooked vegetables.
- Drink approximately one-half ounce of water a day for every pound of body weight. (A 150-pound person, then, would drink about seventy-five ounces of water a day — about nine eight-ounce glasses.)

Those are my general recommendations for a clean diet; they apply both to the next fourteen days and to the rest of your life. The diet you'll be eating over the next fourteen days is designed to energize you and give you dramatic results, and that means:

- no fried foods
- no foods made with refined white flour and/or sugar (cookies, muffins, breads, cakes, most cold cereals, crackers, etc.)
- no energy or power bars or any other packaged, refined, and heavily processed foods
- no gum
- no alcohol

- no dried fruits
- no corn, yams, or potatoes
- no caffeine (no coffee, soda, or caffeinated teas)
- no chocolate
- no artificial sweeteners
- if you're a smoker, you already know that you need to stop; the cardiovascular exercise and increased water consumption will help

Although these are set in stone for the next fourteen days, it wouldn't be a bad idea to eliminate or dramatically reduce these things in your diet forever.

You Can Do It!

Trust me: *you can do this* — even if you've never been able to stick to a diet before, or a workout plan, or a relationship, or piano lessons. This will be different because I'll be with you, every step of the way, coaching and motivating you. You'll have all the information you need to make the choices that have previously been too difficult for you to make for a sustained period of time in the past. You will be strengthened by the WorkOuts you'll be doing and empowered by the WorkIns, and the combination of these mental and physical conditioning exercises will provide you with everything you'll need to change your body, and your life, for good.

Soon these practices will become a part of you, so that you need less and less direction from me, and you'll enjoy more and more variety, choice, and freedom.

You're Not a Cow — Why Are You Grazing?

You'll notice some significant differences between the diet recommendations in Training for Life and some of the popular diets out there. For instance, many people advocate that you eat a bunch of small meals over the course of the day; this is known as "grazing," and I think it's a harmful habit.

When you Train for Life, you *won't* be eating a lot of little meals throughout the day, for a number of reasons. The first has to do with one of our fundamentals: recovery.

Digestion is hard work for the body! It uses *a lot* of energy. When you are constantly asking your body to provide the energy to digest a bunch of mini meals over the course of the day, it takes away from the energy that could be available for other essential processes, processes that aid in weight loss, healing, and maintaining a healthy body. And overtaxing your body's resources will make you look and feel tired.

Eating constantly takes mental energy, too. You're constantly thinking: What have I already eaten today? When can I eat again? What will I have at my next meal? If you're going to live a fuller, and more aware, existence, I'm going to need your mind to focus on more than just food. I want you to eat *appropriately,* not constantly, and in between your meals, you'll find that you have the energy and time to focus on more important things (yes, there are more important things than food), like family, travel, career, and play time.

Your body needs a rest, a real rest, from whatever you have been feeding it lately. That's why *you won't eat during the day* on Day One and Day Eight. Did you just scream, "ARGHHH! Let me out!!"? Keep reading; it's not going to be torture — in fact, once the panic subsides, I think you'll find it quite a serene experience, quieting for both body and mind.

I'm guessing that you've been eating too much, too often, and your poor body has been working overtime just to keep up. That's a great way to look older than your years. And I'd be willing to bet that the foods you've been eating haven't qualified as "clean," either. I want us to start fresh — mentally, emotionally, and physically — so we're going to hit the ground running with a Day One vegetable-broth cleanse. Resting this way helps you get in touch with your body and gain the heightened awareness you need to establish harmony among your mind, body, and food choices. It helps your body work more efficiently, too. Believe me, you won't starve!

No "Bad" Foods

The best thing for me about a clean diet is that it takes so much of the worry out of eating.

Every day I read a new article vilifying one food or another. I laughed out loud when the *New York Times* cited a cholesterol researcher who called the recent panic about trans fats "the panic du jour." That's beautiful, I thought. Government officials and health experts are falling over themselves to condemn these fats (and, often, to replace them with saturated fats), while researchers warn that saturated fats can be equally as dangerous and are four times more prevalent in the average American diet. Is it any wonder that we keep getting fatter and fatter, no matter which panic-du-jour item we cut from our diets?

As far as I'm concerned, all this panicking is another attempt to cheat the system. In truth no donut is really good for you, no matter what kind of fat it's fried in — and no donut is going to kill you either, unless you eat one every day. When you make educated and responsible choices, you don't have to panic; you're insulated from the madness of the moment and immunized against the panic du jour.

You'll eat French fries again — but they're never going to take up enough space in your diet to warrant concern.

Training for Life Nourishes Your Body — And Your Mind!

I can't condition you to like broccoli and to hate chocolate, and I wouldn't want to: you deserve to eat what you like. But I can tell you with confidence that your thoughts, desires, *and actions* will change when you do the healthy mind-body conditioning exercises you'll find in Training for Life. In addition, the menu plans provided will give you the boundaries you need to help redirect and reprogram your eating behaviors.

So eat the meals that I have laid out for you in this book as they are written and commit yourself to the mental and physical practices required of you. This combination will give you a powerful new way of relating to what you eat and how you eat it. And maybe for the first time since childhood, you won't have to spend your days and nights preoccupied by food.

CHAPTER 8

A Fresh Start

"Do away with your old habits and start fresh.

Wash away your old opinions,

and new ideas come in."

—XUE XUAN (1389–1464)

ose weight without exercise!" "Try the new Chocolate, Cheese, and Wine Diet!" "Introducing guilt-free candy, fortified with vitamins and minerals!" "Eat whatever you want, and watch the pounds melt off!"

Why are we always trying to cheat the system? Because that's really what your body is: a system that gains weight when you overeat and don't exercise enough. Whether you know it or not, being overweight, unhealthy, and unfit is a choice that you have made — consciously or unconsciously — over and over again in your life, and that choice has gotten you to where you are today.

Perhaps you can see another road now, life as it could be if you took responsibility for your choices. Are you prepared to choose that road now?

Some of you are ready. You're sick and tired of feeling sick and tired, and it's "go time" for you now. But others of you may be feeling a little trepidation. "Whoa," you think. "My schedule is already stacked; you're asking for a commitment, and I have too many commitments and too little time as it is." You hate working out, and you're unbearable to be around when you're hungry. You're worried you can't give up chocolate — and what are you supposed to do at the movies without popcorn? What if it doesn't work?

In other words you are saying, "I'm not ready."

So maybe you are thinking it would be better to wait and consider this idea again at another time — when a window clears in your schedule, you're feeling more secure at work, or your kids move out. . . .

What you're really saying is "Let's just forget the whole thing."

You're not the first person to have doubts; pretty much everyone I've ever trained has started by saying something very similar. We *all* resist change, especially this kind of change; we gravitate toward what is familiar because breaking out of a pattern is scary. That's OK. You may not feel ready to do this now, but you don't have to feel ready.

You see, I don't need a whole lot to get the ball rolling. I can help you, even when you're not sure of yourself. All I need is a little hope and willingness on your part, and the fact that you're reading this book indicates that you're there. With that small opening I can take you the rest of the way. Eventually your "ready" will kick in, and after fourteen days, you will be capable of taking over from me in the role of coach, believe it or not. But for the next fourteen days, all you have to do is what I have laid out for you in the program, and let the program do the rest.

I'm guessing that you feel stuck, and maybe you've finally hit bottom. I'm not being glib when I say thank goodness that you feel that way and have picked up this book, because your physical, mental, and emotional well-being depend on you making this change NOW. Every day you procrastinate is another day that you won't be enjoying improved health, increased energy, a more vital and youthful appearance, and the other tremendous, multiplying benefits of this practice; instead you will be moving in the opposite direction, as you are right now.

So whether you think you're ready or not, the time to start is now. Now is perfect, now is all there is — so NOW it is. I'm just asking for fourteen days. In that time we will make tremendous progress, even if you feel reluctant and your commitment is weak. Together we will surmount your fears, move past your doubts, rise above your self-imposed limitations, and train like athletes.

I've been on this journey myself. Before I stopped overdrinking and overeating, I thought everybody felt the way I did — blah on a good day and truly terrible on the worst one. My lifestyle (if you can call it that) was slowly killing my body and my spirit. I'd lived like that for so long I didn't know it could be different. First I couldn't see it, and then I couldn't change it. (If you've bought this book, you're already one step ahead of where I started.)

When I'd had enough, I started looking for help, just as you are doing right now. Two things saved me: physical exercise and a personal guide who was with me every step of the way, as I will be with you. These things can save you, too, no matter how scared, desperate, or far gone you think you are. I learned, as you will, to do the mental and emotional conditioning that changed my life for good, and I found that the physical changes were a glorious added benefit — and a necessary one.

Whether you are tired of being overweight and unfulfilled or are looking to completely reinvent yourself; whether you want to move off the plateau you have been stuck on for a while or find yourself curious to see what you're really capable of, these fourteen days will get you where you want to go.

All I need you to do is to answer YES to the following four questions. Read each question and answer it out loud. If you feel comfortable doing so, tell your partner, your family, or a close friend exactly what you intend to do. I have also set up a page on my Web site (www.walkvest.com) so that you may state your intention anonymously to a community at large.

- For the next fourteen days, do you agree to put aside all that you have been "sold" about instant weight loss, miracle cures, and effortless quick fixes?
- Do you accept that you won't be able to change your eating habits or unhealthy lifestyle for any significant amount of time by changing external behaviors — diet and exercise — alone?
- Do you understand that all your thoughts and beliefs inform and support your behaviors and that you cannot effect a long-term change in behavior without fundamentally changing your mind?
- Do you want to live the rest of your life happily and successfully, with peace and ease?

Remember that YES in the context of this program is more than an affirmation of your willingness, it is also a measure of your efforts.

Excellent. Let's begin.

PART TWO

TRAINING FOR LIFE: THE PROGRAM

Phase I

Every day will be governed by one of three fundamentals: **strength, endurance,** or **recovery**. Each day you will be asked to do both a related WorkIn, an exercise to recondition your thoughts and beliefs by repeating a short phrase or sentence over and over during the course of the day, and a WorkOut, your physical training for the day, and to follow a food plan.

I'd like to ask you, as part of your training, to read this book all the way through, cover to cover. The WorkOuts are dense with coaching and advice; it's precisely this coaching that makes this program different from all the others, and I'd like you to get an overall feeling for what I have to say before you begin the fourteen-day program. Please don't worry — you aren't expected to read along with these coaching-intensive WorkOuts as you're working out! You'll find a handy pull-out section at the back of this book that has on it everything you need to remember, including the day's WorkOut, WorkIn, and food plan, and the fuller version will always be here for you to refer back to.

Some of what I ask you to do may seem awkward or trivial, but you must trust me. I wouldn't waste my time developing and writing this program for you (or ask you to waste your time doing it) if I didn't know it would help. So, if only for the next fourteen days, please do what I ask you to do, exactly as I ask you to do it. For instance, some of the first fourteen WorkOuts in this book require that you devote a significant amount of time to exercise. For some of you this time commitment may feel like too much. If that's the case I have a remedy for you — but first let me remind you that these first WorkOuts make up the "boot camp" phase of your training. This phase is designed to give you a powerful foundation for your new, more youthful, more joyful life. Laying this groundwork is the most time-consuming part, but it's also the most invigorating — and the one most likely to reward you with the results you want. Perhaps the commitment I'm asking from you will seem less time-intensive when you consider how these first fourteen days will change you — body and mind — for the rest of your life. Remember: *extraordinary efforts bring extraordinary results.*

That said, we can do important work together at any level of commitment. Don't fall into the trap of waiting until you "have the time," or you'll wait forever. If what I am asking is too much for you to give — even for two weeks — then you must simply pledge to give me your honest and forthright efforts in the time you do have. Figure out how much time you have available each day (mornings, preferably) and reduce each WorkOut by whatever amount of time you must; get going with TFL *now* — even if it means that you stop at the thirty-minute mark each day. For the first fourteen days, I would rather have you do the WalkOut and eliminate the strength, stretch, and tone portion of the WorkOut. No matter how strapped for time you are, please reserve three minutes to cool down. And bear in mind that adding weight to your WorkOuts (in the form of the WalkVest) helps you get the most out of the time you have.

For just fourteen days I'm asking you to suspend what you *think* you can do so that I can show you what I *know* you can do. Make you your number-one priority by putting yourself, your health, and your fitness first.

In the A.M.

- Read each day's plan immediately upon rising if possible — definitely before you begin the juggling act of your morning schedule. Find a private, quiet space in your home in which to read it. (If you're rolling your eyes, stop: I'm asking for just five minutes. And yes, sometimes the only quiet, private space I can find in my own house is behind a locked bathroom door.)

- Sit with a straight spine, close your eyes for a minute, and feel yourself settling into a calm and even breathing pattern. Open your eyes and read your WorkOut and your WorkIn. Then read your WorkIn again, out loud this time. Find a phrase in your WorkIn that you can easily repeat (if not the whole sentence) all day. Write it down; many of my students like to use Post-its so that they can move their WorkIn sentence from the bathroom mirror to the rearview mirror to the computer to the treadmill.

- Use this morning time to decide exactly *when* you will do that day's WorkOut — and to come up with a backup plan, too. For instance, "I will be walking out the door of my office at six p.m., and I will be at the gym by six fifteen." Backup plan: "If something happens to derail that plan, I'll get on my treadmill or go to the gym after the kids go to bed." Anticipate problematic situations and solve them in advance. No time to make lunch? OK — now is the time to figure out what to do instead. Will the cafeteria at work have what you need to stick with the meal plan, or do you have to stop somewhere on the way in to the office this morning?

Respecting this morning ritual is an essential part of the work that you will be doing in the program. This is the time to center yourself, to organize your thoughts and your day, and to reaffirm your commitment to *Training for Life*.

In the P.M.

At the end of every day, before you get into bed, return to the quiet space where your day started and take a few moments to reflect upon your day.

Review the quality of all your efforts over the course of the day: during your Walk-Outs; following the TFL food plan or making food choices; and at work, home, and play. Were your efforts honorable, powerful, and effective? If so you must be feeling a sense of real satisfaction. Notice and enjoy it. If you are dissatisfied, note that feeling, decide how you will do things differently, and let any negative feelings go. You will have another opportunity tomorrow to do your very best.

Allow yourself to get very still and quiet as you say your WorkIn one more time and think about how its meaning has evolved for you since you read it for the first time. Soak in these simple words as you would soak in a hot bath, allowing them to permeate and change every cell of your body. Now that you've absorbed the power of these words, you will always have them; know that you can return to them whenever you need them.

CHAPTER 9

Training Day One: Strength

Stay in the Moment

ur first day of training is a strength day, since physical and mental power will be important right from the very beginning.

Today you will practice *staying in the moment.* Your focus will be on today, and today only. Make a note to your Inner Coach: "Today is the most important day of my training" — as tomorrow will also be tomorrow.

We all have a tendency to distract ourselves from the task at hand. We talk on the phone while we're driving, read the newspaper while eating, watch TV while exercising, and shop online during a conference call. Some people call it multitasking — I call it distraction and avoidance. I know that sometimes it's necessary to do more than one thing at a time, but we too often lose the benefits that would come from fully immersing ourselves in an activity. When we're concentrating on more than one thing, our efforts on the task in front of us are diluted — and our results invariably reflect that lack of focus. Can you really, honestly say that you believe that the workout you get while you're making weekend plans on the phone and watching CNBC represents your purest effort?

As far as I'm concerned, if you're going to expend the energy, you may as well get the most from it. The key, of course, is awareness. *Staying in the moment* increases your awareness and, with it, your ability to focus your energies, which enables you to get better results in less time.

Staying in the moment will make your efforts more effective.

You will see, too, that your tasks seem much less overwhelming if you are fully *in the moment* and focused on what is right in front of you. Doing so allows you to tackle the task in smaller, more manageable bits, instead of trying to grapple with the entirety of it all at once. Imagine standing at the bottom of a hill, looking up at the top; it's discouraging when you can see the full grade of that hill and the distance you'll have to travel. But if you focus instead on just what is immediately in front of you — your next step, as opposed to the top of the hill — the climb doesn't look so steep. And all you have to do is take a single step, the one that's right in front of you.

I read a story once about a former professional wrestler who used to run sprints in the hills. As he ran he'd think, "Short steps; lean forward; don't look too far ahead; short steps; lean forward; don't look too far ahead. " That's not bad advice for *any* kind of uphill struggle!

Staying in the moment prevents us from becoming overwhelmed.

Staying in the moment means being present. Instead of wishing your life away or spending time projecting how life will be *"when"* — recognize each moment as a precious gift. See the present as a *present*, if you will — even if what you're doing is difficult. Because *here* is where you condition yourself, and *here* is where you get better, *here* is where you must live if you want to be truly *alive.*

Today I'll coach you on how to stay in the here and now so that you can deliver a more effectively concentrated effort. You'll reap the rewards of these more potent efforts in faster, and better, results. But you don't need to think about those results today. In fact, don't think at all about the next fourteen days, or next month, or what is to come. Instead concentrate exclusively on your efforts today.

It's *my* job to guide you and to know how worthwhile and effective this training will be for you, in all areas of your life and in the long run. I know that honing your ability to focus and stay in the moment will give you a greater clarity and awareness, which will serve you well beyond your training. But you don't have to concern yourself with any of that; all you need to do now is trust me. Take each task as I give it to you and immerse yourself in it, and that will guarantee your success.

WorkIn: I will stay present in the moment. I will focus my efforts on exactly what I am doing and recognize the present as my gift.

Training for Life Meals

Today our focus is on cleansing your body while still giving it all the nutrients it needs to support its most basic functions.

To do this I want you to put a pot of four to six cups of fresh vegetables and three to five cups of spring water on to boil. Organic is best. Use color as your guide, so that you're including as many different ones as you possibly can: red, orange, purple, yellow, and green.

Here are some suggestions:

Beets
Broccoli
Cabbage (red and white)
Carrots
Cauliflower
Collard greens
Garlic
Green beans
Kale
Mushrooms
Onions
Peppers (red, orange, yellow, green — even spicy varieties)
Shallots
Spinach
Squash
Tomatoes

Simmer for 40 to 60 minutes or until the vegetables are soft. Refrigerate the broth and vegetables separately.

You can season the broth any way you'd like to. One of my students gives it an Asian spin with star anise and ginger; another uses the traditional French bouquet garni (peppercorns, parsley stems, a bay leaf, and a sprig of thyme, all tied together in a piece of cheesecloth). Another one of my students finds that roasting garlic before adding it imparts a sweeter flavor; for another, simple salt and pepper will do. Let your taste guide you to make this recipe your own.

Over the course of the day, you'll drink the broth of this soup, gently warmed on the stovetop or chilled — your preference — I prefer that you don't use a microwave. For your final meal of the day, you'll eat a cup and a half of the vegetables in the soup.

I hope that you'll embrace the challenge of going twelve hours (that's all a day is!) without solid food, but if the thought makes you panic, don't: you may add one-half cup of cooked whole-grain (brown, basmati, or wild) rice two times during the day.

You will also drink fresh spring water; I recommend that you drink eight 8-ounce glasses over the course of the day.

Strength WorkOut

DAY ONE WALKOUT

Note to WalkVest users: please read the instructions that came with your WalkVest thoroughly before using it in your first WalkOut. If you are new to exercise, someone who is recovering from an injury or illness, very unfit, or very overweight, please start exercising with just two pounds in your WalkVest. If you are in relatively good shape already, you can begin with four pounds, or eight weights, evenly distributed. You'll find a utility pocket located in the upper back of your WalkVest for a CD player, your iPod, or your keys.

STEP 1 (1–5 MINUTES):

Warm-up: You'll warm up at the beginning of every WalkOut, moving your way through the Easy Zone of Your Effort Scale (YES).

Walk easily to heat up the muscles in your body. Begin with Your Effort Scale (YES) at 1 and gently increase the intensity of YES to 2, until your body begins to feel warm and your mind more focused.

As you warm up, relax your shoulders as well as your mind. Let everything that doesn't relate directly to these training sessions fall away so that you are able to bring yourself fully to your WorkOut. As you walk, imagine that you are being lifted toward the sky by a thread attached to the top of your head, so that your spine is elongated and your shoulders sit relaxed on your back. Roll your shoulders gently a few times as you walk, shake your hands, wiggle your fingers, and swing your arms comfortably and naturally by your side.

By minute 4 you should feel comfortable increasing YES to 3, and for at least 1 minute, you'll walk tall and secure, knowing that you are entering a very important part of your day — the part where you take care of you by empowering and strengthening every part of who you are.

STEP 2 (6–14 MINUTES):

Over the next 9 minutes, you'll increase your intensity in three 3-minute intervals so that you move through the entire Moderate Zone of Your Effort Scale.

Begin by revving YES from 3 to 4 for the next 3 minutes. You can do this by increasing your walking pace (and your elevation if you are on a treadmill). You should feel a slight but noticeable difference in the deepness of your breath.

After 3 minutes increase your speed and/or elevation again, bringing YES to 5. You're right in the middle of the Moderate Zone. This steady, powerful pace should feel strong, but not strenuous. After 3 minutes here, rev it up to 6, the top level of the Moderate Zone. You're breathing deeply now — not huffing and puffing, but taking air from the bottom of your lungs.

At the same time that you're revving up your physical self, rev your mental self up for an effort that is dedicated and fully aware. You will want to notice everything that is going on — in your body and mind. Notice how your legs feel and how your arm movements change naturally as you increase the pace. Notice how warm your body feels and at what point you begin sweating. As you fine-tune your awareness, you will feel each new level of intensity, no matter how subtle. When you are giving me an effort of 6 on

> **TRAINING TIP**
>
> Lifting up through the top of your head lengthens, strengthens, and opens the spine, which helps create a free flow of energy. It also helps you to walk softly, so you land with a light step, allowing you to float along the road — preserving your joints as you go!
>
> As you walk, be careful not to hit your heel with every footfall. Practice rolling softly from your heel to the ball of your foot, as if you were literally pushing the pavement or treadmill belt behind you. Remind yourself to stay in the moment by concentrating intently on each step, and know that when you land every step softly, you're training compassionately.

YES, you will know it by the strength and energy you feel in your breath and in your heart.

STEP 3 (15–19 MINUTES):

Turn the volume on your efforts *down* to 4 on YES over the next 5 minutes. Gradually decrease your speed and elevation so you move through YES 6 to 5 to a less intense effort of 4. This is the low end of your Moderate Zone; we are not going back to Easy just yet, but 4 should satisfy your need to recover.

STEP 4 (20–25 MINUTES):

Now you'll increase YES from 4 into the YES Power Zone by increasing your pace (and the incline of your treadmill) for three 2-minute increments. As you move from 4 to 5 to 6 to 7, use the full 2 minutes at each new level of intensity to adjust and appreciate the way your body feels at this new level. At 6 you're working at the top of YES's

TRAINING TIP

Your abs aren't just there to make you miserable during bathing suit season; they make up a significant portion of the muscles at the core of your body, the muscles that keep you upright. Strengthening these core muscles improves your posture, helps reduce your chance of injury, and strengthens and protects your lower back.

So draw your abdominal muscles in toward your spine as you walk and make sure that you don't collapse into that core. It's a good way to get the physical stability you'll need and provides you with a balanced and safe stride.

Ultimately this conditioning will strengthen and tighten your abs, leaving you with a flatter tummy. And of course the conditioning we're doing here also strengthens your mental core, by laying a strong foundation for the practices to come.

Moderate Zone, so your breathing will become very deep, although you will try to keep it steady and even. At 7 you're entering the Power Zone, which will require you to give more effort, more energy, and a more passionate commitment. *Dig in* as you break a new barrier.

Stay at 7 for 2 minutes and swing your arms to generate the intensified effort, increased heart rate, and elevated energy expenditure that I am asking for. Staying in the present moment means being in touch with *all* of the changes, whether subtle or strong, pleasant or uncomfortable, that are happening in your body and mind.

Note to Your Inner Coach

Staying Strong in the Moment: The Mind-Body Check-In

It takes a great deal of discipline to stay totally focused. I'm human, too, and sometimes I find my mind drifting away from my efforts during my WorkOuts. "How will I talk the kids out of their favorite restaurant tonight — and into going anywhere *but* there?" I wonder. "Why, when we have the technology to fly, do our cars still roll on the ground?"

Spacing out happens, even though we all know that getting totally fit is truly a combined effort between our minds and our bodies. I often find that the answer is to reaffirm the connection between the two: checking in with myself *physically* focuses and calms my mind and helps return my attention to the task at hand.

Here are some of the questions you might ask yourself in order to help you get back in the moment:

• Are you breathing comfortably or stressfully? Your breath is a great source of energy. Is your breathing appropriate for the level of effort you are supposed to be giving? If I find that my breathing is stressful during my warm-up, for instance, I'll slow my pace and give my body a chance to get back into the Easy Zone.

• Are you walking tall and proud? Have your shoulders crept up around your ears? Is your chest open? Are your abs engaged and strong so they support your lower back?

• Are you walking lightly, hitting the treadmill belt or pavement softly? Are you rolling off the ball of your foot, pushing the ground purposefully behind you, while still maintaining a comfortable and natural stride?

• Are you holding tension in your body? For instance, are your hands clenched? Is your jaw set and tight? Is your brow furrowed? If so, let go.

Once you've reestablished yourself physically, repeat your WorkIn to yourself. I call this my **mind-body check-in**. Running through this physical checklist helps me to reconnect my mind with what's happening in my body and to return my focus to what I'm doing — at least until the next time I drift again. . . . "Should I adopt another dog?"

STEP 5 (26–30 MINUTES):

Decrease your walking speed, a little at a time, back to 5 on YES. Although you are still in the Moderate Zone and still moving forward with a dutiful effort, there should be an obvious feeling of recovery and relief in this 5-minute interval. Feel how grateful your body is for the respite.

STEP 6 (31–34 MINUTES):

From a YES of 5, increase your pace and elevation to a YES 6 for 2 minutes, and then again to 7 for 2 minutes. Here you must focus your energies intently to avoid distraction. Increasing intensity from a place of recovery is difficult at first for most of us; it takes a diligent and strong-hearted effort, and the *only* way that I know to get that effort is to be present in each moment.

STEP 7 (35–36 MINUTES):

It's time to take it to another level: hit it. We'll do this for just two short intervals.

Take YES to 8, engaging your upper and lower body, as well as your intellect and your passion. Swing your arms powerfully and stay there for 1 minute — just 60 seconds! As your breathing becomes more stressful, you may notice that you begin to doubt your abilities. You may hear a familiar voice second-guessing your intentions, and there may even be a

TRAINING TIP

You'll be surprised to notice the relief you get from even a slight reduction in pace; that's the miracle of these recovery periods. But bear in mind that it should never be so much of a cutback that it feels like you are on a break!

The goal is to stay just as aware, prepared, and focused on the present moment while in the recovery intervals as you do during the intensity intervals. That way, your mind and body work in unison under all circumstances and conditions — and in recovery *all of you* gets the breather you need.

TRAINING TIP

Keep your arms, your shoulders, and your hands relaxed, even as you begin to use them to increase Your Effort Scale. When you tense up, you steal necessary energy from yourself — energy that could be going directly into your training.

brief moment of fear of failure (or success). This is to be expected, if you are giving the effort that I am asking of you; in fact, it's actually a good sign — it means that you are paying attention! Don't worry; you have all the coaching, motivation, and support you'll need to help you break through to a whole new level.

And, when that first minute is up, you're going to hit it harder, taking

> **TRAINING TIP**
>
> Swinging your arms to help drive your walking speed and heart rate up has another benefit: it sculpts, tones, and strengthens all the muscles in your upper body, including those in your arms, chest, shoulders, and back.

YES to 9 for 1 minute. You're reaching the top of Your Effort Scale here, and you need all the energy and attention you can bring to it, so focus only on what is happening *right now, in this moment.* You'll know you've reached the desired level of intensity when you find yourself saying, "I don't think I've ever given this much before." Give me the strongest, purest, most focused 9 you can muster!

This powerful effort made by you, *for* you, will shape your spirit as it shapes your body and strengthens your heart. It will provide you with the ability to dig deep inside and hit it whenever you need to.

STEP 8 (37–41 MINUTES):

Level I: Beginners
Level II: Intermediate to Advanced

Here is your first chance to coach yourself. Have you had enough? Do you think a 3-minute recovery interval will give you what you need to continue, as Level II Training for Lifers will? Then go on to Level II instructions. Have you given me everything you've got, leaving you ready for some R&R? (When you train for life, R&R stands for rest and reflect, incidentally.) Then follow directions for Level I.

Choose wisely. Be cautiously aggressive with your efforts: don't go too far too soon, but certainly don't cheat yourself out of the powerful WorkOut that you are capable of.

DAY ONE STRENGTH WORKOUT

Level I (37–41 minutes):

Go to the R&R box below.

Level II (37–39 minutes):

Decrease your walking speed and Your Effort Scale to 4, little by little, in this quick, 3-minute recovery interval. With only 3 minutes to recover, you must *key in* mentally to your body's recovery — use your head to guide your heart. When your mind and body work together, you get the most effective and productive intensity and recovery periods.

STEP 9
Level II (40–43 minutes):

Rev it back up, from YES 5 to 6, and then 6 to 7, staying at each level for 2 minutes.

STEP 10
Level II (44–45 minutes):

Get into your Power Zone and hit 8 on YES for 1 minute and then 9 for 1 minute more. Maintain your composure and posture in both your mind and your body and stay present in every feeling, every breath, and every thought. This may be a difficult moment to stay in, but you will benefit from the effort.

STEP 11
Level II (46–50 minutes):

It's your turn to rest and reflect: go to the R&R box below.

REST AND REFLECT

Stay in the Moment — *All* the Way

This is your final recovery period. Dial YES back gradually over the next 5 minutes, all the way back to 1, so that in your last minute or 2 or 3, you are walking in your Easy Zone. Use this time to reflect on how your body feels

---

right now, given the work you've done today. Keep your stride, posture, and awareness intact as you step lightly, easily, all the way home.

The final few moments of every WalkOut will always be dedicated to rest and reflection. Although this portion of the WalkOut may be physically easier than the rest of it, it's very important that you stay as focused here as you are during every other part of the WalkOut and work *precisely* in every moment. It's easy to relax our purposefulness and get distracted at the very end of a WalkOut — or indeed, at the end of any task; we're tired and ready to be done. But compromising your commitment to *staying in the moment* in these last seconds is a waste, and self-destructive, too.

Don't give in to your old ways. Honor yourself and your efforts by staying present to the very last stride, and respect your recovery by giving it the same respect that you give the rest of your WorkOut. Trust me, you're not too tired to make these final efforts as pure and diligent as the ones that came before.

Stretch, Strengthen, and Tone (approximately 10 minutes)

If you're wearing a WalkVest, remove it.

If it's too uncomfortable to get down on the floor for these exercises, DON'T do them. DO stay committed to your WalkOuts, though, and soon you will be strong enough, lean enough, and agile enough to join us.

FULL REST

Lie flat on your stomach on a soft surface (a mat, carpeting, or a patch of grass), with your head turned to one side. Relax your body completely, letting it melt into the ground. Let your shoulders fall forward as your neck relaxes and feel your arms sink heavily into the earth. Notice how everything feels — your breath, the surface you are lying on, the weight of your legs, your neck, and your cheek against the ground. *Don't fall asleep!* You must be awake to be aware. After 30 seconds, turn your head to the other side. Stay very still for 30 seconds more as you release your body completely.

PUSH-UPS

Today, we're going to do a few sets of push-ups. These exercises are fantastic for the arms and chest, and keeping your core muscles solid will also help to tone your middle.

There are a number of different ways to do push-ups.

- **The classic:** In this position, your weight is on your hands and the balls of your feet. If you choose to do your push-ups this way, keep your core engaged and your rear end down, in line with your shoulders, as

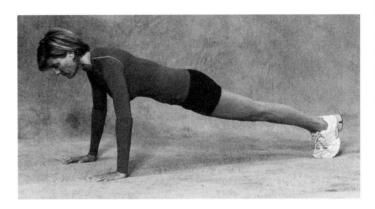

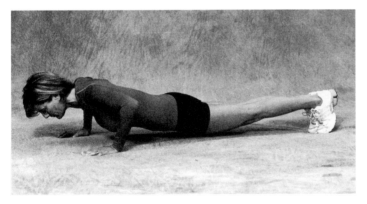

though you were a solid plank of wood, from head to toe. Your back shouldn't arch, nor should your butt stick up into the air.

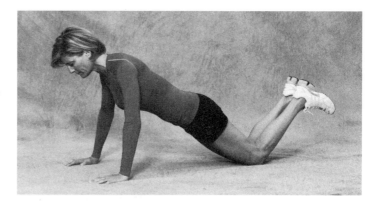

- **Bent knees:** You can do the classic push-up with your knees bent and on the ground. This is a slightly easier version

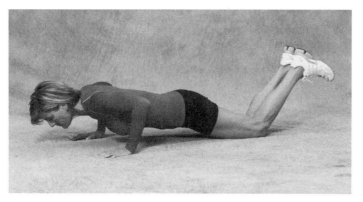

than the classic way, but doing them this way will still help you to build upper body strength.

- **With leverage:** Assume the classic push-up position with your hands slightly elevated (on the first step of a staircase, for instance). This will make the push-ups easier; the

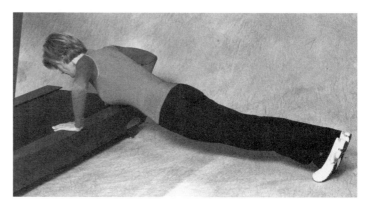

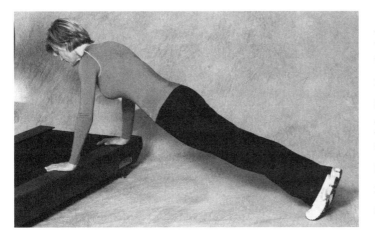

higher the step, the easier the push-up. If you want to make the push-ups harder, assume the classic push-up position with your *feet* slightly elevated (on the first step of a staircase, for instance). The higher the step, the harder the push-up.

No matter what position you choose, your hands should be evenly placed, a little wider than shoulder-width apart, and flat on the floor. Your abs should be engaged, and your eyes should be on the floor just slightly in front of you; but don't crane your neck.

On an inhale, slowly bend your arms and lower yourself to an inch or two off the floor; as you exhale, imagine pushing the floor away with your breath, straighten your arms, and push yourself back up. Count 2 on the way up and 2 on the way down, and keep your core muscles engaged throughout the exercise.

> ### TRAINING TIP
>
> NEVER sacrifice form for level of difficulty. Choose the position that works best for you, allowing you to complete the sets and repetitions required. If you compromise the integrity of this or any exercise, you condition yourself to do the work incorrectly, which runs contrary to everything that we are trying to accomplish; it also puts you at greater risk of injury.

Level I:

Do 3 sets of 5 repetitions each.

Level II:

Do 3 sets of 8 repetitions each.

CHEST LIFT

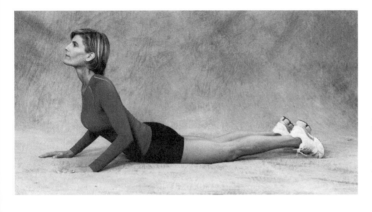

Put your hands flat on the floor in line with your chest on either side of your body. Keep your hips and pelvis in contact with the floor and lift your head off the floor, looking straight ahead of you, as you gently press your shoulders and chest up off the floor. If you feel comfortable raise your gaze toward the sky. Arch your back, but don't compress in the lower spine; instead imagine your torso getting longer as you extend out through the chest. Shoulders should be relaxed, down and back.

Hold this position for 10 seconds and then slowly lower your upper body back to the floor with your head turned to one side. Relax there for 10 seconds and repeat. Alternate the side on which you rest your head.

This is great toning for your shoulders and arms and a beautiful stretch for your chest, hip flexors, and mid torso. As you lift, feel the opening that you create in your chest when you do this exercise.

SINGLE KNEE HUG

Roll over onto your back and lie flat, again letting your whole body — especially your lower back and shoulders — melt into the floor. Keeping your hips even and your lower back in contact with the ground, if possible, bend one leg and bring it into your

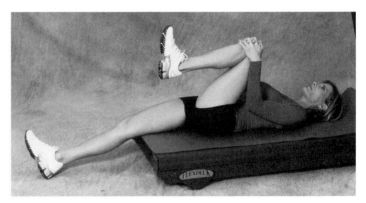

chest. You may need to use a strap (a belt, a tie, or a towel will work) to extend your reach. Clasp your hands together two inches below the kneecap and hug the knee into your body.

Be cautious *not* to tense up your upper body — keep your shoulders and neck relaxed, with your head on the ground, while holding the knee and hugging it in toward your chest. Keeping your head on the floor, tilt your chin down ever so slightly and look toward your knee without straining. This helps straighten and elongate the spine.

Do not let go and drop your leg to the floor, but release slowly after holding for 10 seconds. Do this 2 more times (holding for 10 seconds each) on each side, seeing if you feel a little more flexible on the second and third attempts.

CRUNCHES

Lie on your back, with your knees bent, feet on the floor. You can hook your feet under the couch or a sturdy chair or have your workout partner hold them. Place your hands on your opposite shoulders, so that your arms are crossed in an X across your chest. Keeping your chin tucked into your chest, contract your abs and bring your upper back off the floor about six inches; hold your body in the crunch for 2 counts (say it out loud: up, one, two, down). Make sure to intensify the contraction of your abs by pulling them in toward your spine while you're in the crunch.

Level I:
2 sets of 8.

Level II:
3 sets of 10.

CHEST LIFT

Finally, roll over on your belly one last time and do one very slow chest lift for a full abdominal stretch.

TRANQUILITY POSE

Slowly get up, and stand tall. With deliberation reach your arms away from your sides and up to the sky, pressing your palms and fingers together over your head. Stretch your upper body away from your lower body by reaching your fingertips to the sky and see if you

can feel new spaces in your back, your shoulders, your armpits, and your rib cage. Keep your chin level to the floor — and, as we do while walking, imagine that a silver thread is lifting you, crown first, to the sky. Hold this stretch for a count of 5 and release by bringing your palms — still pressed together — straight down in front of you by bending both elbows so that your palms pass in front of your face slowly and rest at your heart center.

Now, with eyes closed or open, be still, be calm, and *be* in the moment. Breathe, relax, surrender, and relinquish any tension that you may still have. Hold for a count of 10 (at least), then release.

Be mindful in every moment of your day today.

CHAPTER 10

Training Day Two: Endurance

Handle with Care

I t simply isn't enough for someone to tell you that you are valuable, or beautiful, or intelligent, or even that you're loved. For any of these qualities to make a difference in our lives, we must believe it ourselves. Today you are going to think about whether *you* consider yourself valuable — and whether you do or not, today's WorkIn is going to help you fortify the belief that you *are*.

We treat our valuable treasures with care. We hold a new baby as if just breathing on her will break her; our family heirlooms are insured and rest in a safe-deposit box; the new car gets a weekly wash and wax and sleeps in the garage, protected from vandals and weather. Taking good care of something is how we show that we consider it to be valuable. So what does it say about our opinions of ourselves when we consistently overeat — not to mention engaging in other self-destructive behaviors, such as smoking and regularly drinking too much? We can really only draw the conclusion that a person who engages in that kind of behavior doesn't think much of herself at all.

This can be an unsettling realization. You may not *think* you feel unworthy — because feelings and beliefs reside at conscious and subconscious levels. But our actions don't lie. Many of us confuse pride in our achievements, accomplishments, and possessions with a true feeling of self-worth. Consciously you may be proud of yourself — for the career you've developed, the kids you've raised, the friendships you've maintained, and the home you've created. Maybe you're a fabulous cook, or a brilliant investor, or an accomplished artist; these are all things to be proud of. But being proud of what you *do* and what you *have* is not the same thing as valuing who you *are*.

Your personal value is not now and never has been based on what you do or what you have. Your individual worth as a person is not based on what others think of you, your IQ, your position at work, or the amount of money in your bank account. You may be proud of all those things, and they certainly have value in your life, but as long as you are engaging in self-destructive thoughts and behaviors, you are indicating that you don't feel worthy of better care. By the way, your value is not based on your weight either — or the size of your thighs or your waistline.

I wish that I had a way to state this more emphatically, but all I have at the moment are these words, so let me tell you the glorious truth: no matter who you are, what you do, where you come from, or what you have, **you are valuable.**

It's time you started believing it so you can start acting like it. You must feel worthy of better care so that you will take better care of yourself more consistently. This is why reconditioning your thoughts about yourself through the TFL WorkIns is so important. Choosing to participate in Training for Life is part of making a *valuable* investment in yourself and is a true expression of self-care. When you believe (truly believe, as the WorkIns will help you to do) that you are valuable in your own right, you will be able to make healthful choices more easily and more often. When you behave as if you are worthy of all the blessings that you have, as well as those you desire, you'll know ease and happiness like never before. And losing weight will be just a small part of your total fitness transformation.

WorkIn: **I am valuable. I treat myself with care, love, and respect. My worth as a person is nonnegotiable.**

Training for Life Meals

Breakfast: one-half grapefruit, one or two soft-boiled/poached eggs, three tomato slices, and five cucumber slices.

Lunch: one cup or can of soup and two cups of fresh salad, sprinkled with dressing. One slice of whole-grain (wheat free if possible) bread or toast, no butter.

Dinner: four to six ounces baked/grilled fish (salmon, tuna, halibut) or chicken breast, seasoned to taste. One cup of salad or gently cooked vegetables of your choice.

Snacks: ten fresh, raw, unsalted almonds and one-half cup blueberries.

Over the course of the day, drink eight 8-ounce glasses of water.

Endurance WorkOut

DAY TWO WALKOUT

STEP 1 (1–5 MINUTES):

Warm-up: Walk easily, starting with Your Effort Scale at 1 to warm up your body. Relax your shoulders and remember to lift gently out of the top of your head, so that you are walking tall and stepping lightly. Your arms should be comfortably relaxed by your side as you gradually walk through the YES Easy Zone.

STEP 2 (6–20 MINUTES):

You'll be doing 3 sets of increasingly intense intervals, 5 minutes each. Five minutes is a pretty long interval, so it's important to make sure that you carefully monitor Your Effort Scale. Don't give too much too soon and don't drift away, mentally or physically. Keep your focus intact by noticing what happens as you walk: the speed and sound of your breathing, the heat of your body, and even what's going on with your facial muscles. Are you walking around with a grimace or a smile? A smile is better.

Walk for 5 minutes at YES 4. Then increase your pace to YES 5 and walk there for 5 minutes, keeping the same level of awareness. Increase your exercise intensity again, this time to 6 — the top of the Moderate Zone — for 5 minutes. As the intensity of your WalkOut escalates, repeat with increasing enthusiasm your WorkIn for today: "I am valuable!"

Note to Inner Coach

Get Out of Your Own Way

When I tell my students to swing their arms for the first time, they inevitably swing them across their body. In this way they cut themselves off — literally getting in their own way — instead of propelling themselves forward.

How many times in life do we unconsciously (or consciously) interfere with our own progress? Is it sabotage, an unconscious belief that we are unworthy, or just misguided instincts? Probably some or all of the above. But when you believe that you are valuable, your behavior supports your health, promotes your progress, and protects your happiness; when you don't, you work against yourself in ways both big and small.

We may not be able to eliminate these behaviors altogether, but we can certainly stay aware of them, stop them when we notice them, and make a conscious effort to support our improvement and evolution instead of interfering with our progress.

STEP 3 (21–25 MINUTES):

Turn *down* YES to 4. The reduction in intensity will allow you to recover, building your endurance. Walk at this moderately strong pace — no loafing here — and stay focused on what you are doing. Notice how long it takes you to catch your breath and how difficult or easy it is for you to intensify again when it is time to do that. All of this is *valuable* information for you and will quickly build you a powerful fitness future.

It is as important to train your body (especially your heart) to recover efficiently as it is to lose weight, build muscle, and build bone strength. Reaffirm for yourself that you are worthy of effective and compassionate training: *you deserve to train wisely.*

Note to Your Inner Coach

To value yourself is to value your resources, and your energy is one of the most valuable resources you have. Training compassionately by allowing yourself time to recover allows you to take better care of yourself and shows that you value your resources by using them wisely.

STEP 4 (26–35 MINUTES):

Over the next 10 minutes, you will escalate YES from 5 to 8. Intervals will be shorter and more intense as you get closer to the finish line. Increase your intensity by increasing your pace (and the incline of your treadmill, if you're on one) and walk, for the first 4 minutes, with YES at 5. Get your speed up enough so that you feel strong in your efforts but not overly taxed.

Next increase your intensity to 6 and walk for 3 minutes, then 2 minutes on 7, and one minute at 8. You're in your Power Zone now; push and roll off the ball of your foot and swing your arms. That way you'll effectively use your upper- and lower-body muscles to create powerful momentum. Remember to keep the integrity of your walking form intact as the intensity rises. And above all, remember that you are worthy of your finest efforts.

Note to Your Inner Coach

I know you've heard the saying that "you are what you eat." Guess what? You are how you train, too. If you walk with poise and confidence, chances are good that you will act with poise and confidence in the rest of your life as well — and if you slump, resist, and spend your WalkOut looking for ways to cut corners, that unimpressive attitude is going to carry itself out into the rest of your life as well. Train yourself to give a level of effort that represents you proudly.

STEP 5 (36–40 MINUTES):

Turn *down* YES to 5 in your Moderate Zone, recognizing that even this small step down in intensity offers you the opportunity to recover while you continue training at very high levels of efficiency. In training, as in life, everything is relative, and YES 5 now feels like a welcome break, doesn't it? Stay focused and very present in your WorkOut — do not drop YES below 5 for the next 5 minutes.

STEP 6 (41–52 MINUTES):

Dial up your effort by increasing your speed and incline (if using a treadmill) to YES 6 for 5 minutes, gently moving to the top of your Moderate Zone. Then 7 for 4 minutes, carefully managing your entrance into the Power Zone, and then YES 8 for 3 minutes.

STEP 7 (53–57 MINUTES):

Walk for 5 minutes at YES 5. Walk with pride, a moderately powerful stride, and appreciate this time to recover. Sufficient recovery is the key to long-term success at *everything*.

STEP 8

Level I (58–62 minutes):

Great job! Go to the R&R Box opposite.

Level II (58–60 minutes):

For 3 minutes reduce YES from 5 to 4 and walk lightly, relaxing your upper body by rolling your shoulders. As your body gets used to the recovery process, you will do it more effectively so that you get more out of it in less time.

STEP 9

Level II (61–68 minutes):

Go directly to 6 on Your Effort Scale and WalkOut for 4 minutes. Your abs are engaged, your shoulders are down, your spine is long, and your arms should begin to pump harder now in order to drive the level of intensity up.

After 4 minutes at 6, intensify your efforts slightly, and go to 7 on YES for 4 minutes.

TRAINING TIP

Fatigue is as much mental as it is physical. Sometimes your mind will tell you you're tired when your body has lots more to give.

Don't sell yourself short; have the same faith in yourself that I have in you. Repeat your WorkIn and see if you can keep moving forward dutifully and break through barriers — both mental and physical. Doing this will give you powerful new evidence of the value of this training, and it will confirm your faith in your new ability to move beyond the places you've been stuck before.

This is endurance training; give me your honest-to-goodness best because *nothing* is more valuable than your best effort.

STEP 10
Level II (69–73 minutes):
Go to the R&R box below.

REST AND REFLECT

Reduce YES little by little, all the way back to 1, and walk slowly until your breathing, your body, and your sense of humor has fully recovered. Continue to walk at a relaxed pace for a full 5 minutes.

Slowly roll your shoulders back a few times and then forward a few times. Shake your arms as they hang by your sides and wiggle your fingers as you enjoy the last few moments of your WalkOut. Walk poised, elongated, and proud all the way home. You've given a beautiful and valuable performance. Brilliant work!

Today we worked on elevating your conscious awareness, especially related to your own value. This awareness has benefits that extend beyond the obvious — for example, the way you impact those around you, especially the people who love you. Your low self-esteem and poor health has a seriously detrimental effect on people close to you, whether you realize it or not. When you don't care for yourself, you are not fully available to care well for others — and that *is* selfish. So if anyone tells you that taking time for your own self-improvement is selfish, don't buy it; there's nothing more important than you taking care of you. Set a good example by taking good care of yourself.

It's time to do some stretching and floor work.

Stretch and Abs (approximately 5 minutes)

If you are wearing a WalkVest, remove it and lie flat on your stomach on a soft surface with your head turned to one side.

FULL REST (SEE PAGE 78)

SINGLE KNEE HUG (SEE PAGE 82)

Repeat 2 times on each side.

CRUNCHES (SEE PAGE 83)

Level I:
3 sets of 6.

Level II:
3 sets of 10.

TRANQUILITY POSE (SEE PAGE 84)

Have a priceless day.

CHAPTER 11

Training Day Three: Recovery

Recover on the Road

We've all had days, weeks, and months that are jam-packed with appointments and commitments and things to remember under penalty of death. Maybe your whole life feels that way. You probably think that something radical has to happen for this to change: maybe your kids will move out or you'll win the lottery so you can quit your job and hire a team of full-time assistants.

In fact, you can keep your kids and your job (sorry!), and although I strongly encourage you to get help whenever it's feasible, you don't need to hire anyone. All you need to do is learn to *recover on the road.*

This concept is especially important for those of us with super-busy schedules. With practice you'll discover that even the craziest, most nonstop days present you with many valuable opportunities to recover — you just have to know where to look.

I know you're thinking easier said than done, right? You've been told by your doctors, your children, your shrink, and your kids' shrink that you need to chill out, but you still go, go, go until you're totally depleted. You've read all the books on ways to relax and listened to meditation tapes, but you still can't seem to slow down.

This time things will be different, because Training for Life is different. The intensity of your WorkOuts, and the efficiency with which I want your body (and mind) to operate, means that I *must* give you ample time to recover during your WorkOuts so that you can work to your full potential and stay safe and strong throughout. You'll learn how to apply this principle in your daily life. This way you will get the very most out of everything you do, and you'll feel super — not spent — at the end of every WorkOut and at the end of every day.

Sometimes all it takes to recover is just learning to switch from high gear to a lower one for a little while. Training for Life can teach you how to go from multitasking at sixty miles an hour in service of your various bosses to finding five or ten minutes of peace and quiet just for you. If you spend most of your day with children, ten minutes of adult conversation or reading the newspaper can be a real respite. If your days are spent staring at a computer terminal under fluorescent lighting, then consider *taking it outside* for ten minutes; a short walk in the fresh air will clear your head and lift your spirits. Lock yourself in the bathroom for a short bath while your best friend takes over with the kids. Learn to use the "do not disturb" sign on your office door or just turn off the lights/computer/phone/pager/television and sit, without doing anything at all.

In order to make these changes, you need to understand how destructive your "going, going, gone" behavior really is. You may have been conditioned to believe that it's noble for you to do for others at your own expense, but that's short-term thinking. You're no good to your boss if you're home sick, you're no good to your kids if you're frazzled from not having enough time for yourself, and you'll be no good to anyone once you've run yourself into the ground.

It's time to recognize this behavior for what it is: self-sabotage and an excuse for staying exactly where you are. Recovery is an important part of caring for yourself, and caring for yourself is absolutely essential if you want to take good care of anyone else. Learning to change the way you think and the way you take care of yourself takes physical and mental conditioning, and *that* is what Training for Life excels at, so the changes that occur won't be just momentary, but lifelong.

Since this is Training for Life, we need to be realistic. What will you do when you find (as you inevitably will) that you're fading because you've neglected to recover adequately on any given day or week? Look at your calendar and ask yourself where you might be able to make up a little recovery time — soon. Cancel a social event, say no to one of the little extra obligations you tend to pick up along the way, or ask someone to cover for you while you sleep a little late, go to bed a little early, or take an hour just for yourself.

Most of the time, I know, you demand a lot from yourself. But today I want you to pay close attention to how you feel throughout the day and to what you *need* in order to feel better. When you find yourself feeling tired or moody, look for, and seize, an opportunity to recover and recharge. Give yourself — and your family, your friends, and your career — this very important gift of self-care.

Note to Your Inner Coach

I'd like to talk for a minute about the concept of "stuffing."

We all do it. We load our plates at the buffet, we cram a trip to the cleaners or the market into the ten minutes between appointments. Even our kids run nonstop between school, guitar lessons, soccer practice, and ceramics.

I think this stuffing is one of the most unhealthy things we do to ourselves because it means there's no chance to recover. So unless it's Thanksgiving and you're talking about the turkey — *don't do it.* Don't stuff your day, don't stuff your kids' days, don't stuff your plate, and don't stuff your face. It may sound a little glib, but what I'm really talking about is finding the balance between "enough" and "too much."

Think about that run to the market during a break on a busy day. "It's so efficient!" we tell ourselves. But leaving yourself with no recovery time is anything *but* efficient in the long run; better to sit down and read the paper with a cup of tea for fifteen minutes and rejuvenate yourself for the afternoon ahead. When you fill every second of your day, you become a human doing, not a human being — and when you stop, you'll be able to *feel* more, *notice* more, and take better care of yourself.

The same thing goes for food. Overeating is just a way to numb yourself; the only things you feel when you're stuffed are guilt and shame. That's not nourishment or enjoyment — it's just too much. When you stop overeating, you'll be able to feel what's really going on inside, and then you can begin to change.

So when it comes to workouts, meals, and our daily activities, let's agree to *not* stuff. No overtraining or overworking and no overloading our plates or our days.

WorkIn: Recovery is a necessity, not a luxury. I will pay close attention to how I am feeling, inside and out, and I will find ways to recover when I need to.

Training for Life Meals

Breakfast: two-thirds cup berries (strawberries/blueberries/raspberries) with one-half cup of low-fat or nonfat yogurt or cottage cheese and ten almonds.

Lunch: bunless chicken, turkey, soy, or veggie burger topped with lettuce and tomato, ketchup (one-half tablespoon), and/or mustard. One cup of vegetable/lentil soup or steamed veggies.

Dinner: stir-fry. Toss two cups of freshly cut vegetables into a very hot wok or deep pan with one tablespoon of oil. Stir-fry for a few moments with a little salt and pepper, garlic, tamari, or white wine and serve on top of one-half cup whole-grain brown rice, basmati rice, millet, or quinoa.

Snacks: one grapefruit and one papaya.

Over the course of the day, drink eight 8-ounce glasses of water.

> ### TRAINING TIP
>
> When it comes to selecting vegetables, remember that variety is key: yellow and green squashes; zucchini; mushrooms; cabbage; broccoli; green, yellow, or red peppers; carrots; celery; bean sprouts are all good.

Recovery WorkOut

DAY THREE WALKOUT

STEP 1 (1–5 MINUTES):

Warm-up: Walk easily to warm up your body, going from YES 1 to 3 during these first 5 minutes of your WalkOut.

Right from the start make the connection between your body and your mind. When you walk tall, you walk proud, and when you step lightly, you make progress with a light heart. Use these first few moments of your training to agree to pledge to give a worthy and honorable effort throughout.

STEP 2 (6–20 MINUTES):

For the next 15 minutes, you'll build your exercise intensity gently and slowly, in 3 increments of 5 minutes each.

First increase the intensity of your efforts from YES 3 to YES 4 and stay there for 5 minutes. Luxuriate in the feeling of the work as you move from the top of the Easy Zone to the lowest level of your Moderate Zone.

Increase your efforts again, bringing YES to 5, and stay there for 5 minutes. Since you'll be moving a little more slowly today, take the time to fine-tune the awareness of your physical form: your posture, the way your foot hits the ground.

Move to YES 6 for the last 5 minutes of this period. This is the top end of your Moderate Training Zone, but it shouldn't feel taxing. Walk with a powerful, relaxed pace.

TRAINING TIP

If it takes you longer than 5 minutes to get really well warmed up, then *take it!* The time suggestions I give here are merely recommendations based on my experience and expertise and are my best guess about what *you* need. Soon you (and your Inner Coach) will know even better than I do about what your body needs on any given day, and I hope you'll heed your personal cues.

The same goes for the time recommendations throughout. These numbers are an estimate, designed to give you a guideline for how long these intervals should take. They may not be perfect, but your best efforts are.

Note to Your Inner Coach

A Contradiction in Terms

You may have noticed that I sometimes use what seem to be conflicting adjectives to describe what I'd like you to be feeling or doing. For instance, I might ask you to move "with a powerful but relaxed pace," and you may be wondering whether that isn't a contradiction in terms, like "jumbo shrimp."

In fact I'm purposely using these seemingly opposite concepts to give you an opportunity to see things — even exercise — differently.

"Power" and "relaxation" need not be mutually exclusive; in fact they complement each other, and embracing both of them simultaneously will actually enhance your experience. A strong effort doesn't have to put strain on your body and mind; indeed, it shouldn't! Learning to give effort with ease allows you to stay on the road and to enjoy the journey.

STEP 3 (21–25 MINUTES):

Reduce your intensity, from YES 6 to YES 4. Relax and walk with greater ease for 5 minutes.

Note to Inner Coach

Getting the Most Out of Your Recovery

You can't expect to look or feel your best if you haven't had sufficient recovery time. That's one reason that it's so important to intersperse these Recovery Training Days among your Strength and Endurance Training Days.

Since recovery days require less from you *physically*, they give you an opportunity to turn your concentration more powerfully inward. They allow us the time and space to reinforce the positive habits and techniques, like the mind-body check-ins, that allow us to feel young, strong, and vital, no matter what we're coping with.

These habits can be hard to remember when the days are long and difficult — we're too focused on the finish line. So use your recovery days wisely, to condition yourself to recover and to make that habit so deeply ingrained that it's always at hand when you need it.

STEP 4 (26–35 MINUTES):
Upper-Body WorkOut: The Pyramid (arms, shoulders, chest, back)

Over the next 10 minutes, we're going to add some upper-body exercises that will not only tone, stretch, and strengthen your upper body but also increase the cardiovascular intensity of your WalkOut.

Modify your walking pace so that Your Effort Scale stays at 4. Remind yourself that today is all about recovery, even though there is work to be done.

Bring both arms up so that your elbows are at shoulder height and bent at right angles. I call this the "field-goal" position.

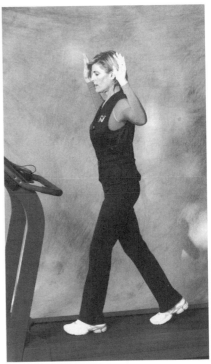

From your field-goal position, straighten your arms for a count of 5 and reach for the sky so that your fingertips meet over your head, stretching up and holding for a count of 1. With control, take 5 counts to lower your arms back to field-goal position, so that your upper arms are parallel to the ground and your forearms are perpendicular to it.

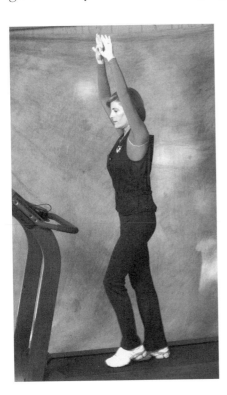

While your arms are in the field-goal position, bring your elbows back so that they're slightly behind the shoulders. Then reach away from your body with each elbow to stretch the chest and back and upper arms, as though someone were pulling your bent arms east and west away from your torso. This will open your chest and give you a nice stretch in the upper arms and shoulders.

Over the next 10 minutes, Level I will do 4 sets of 6 repetitions each; Level II will do 4 sets with 12 repetitions each. After each set, recover your upper-body strength and comfort by releasing your arms to your side and shaking them out from shoulders to fingertips. Roll the shoulders back a few times and continue on with your walk, feeling the relief and pleasure of both the exercise and the rest. Take a nice break (about 60 seconds or so) in between each set.

STEP 5 (36–40 MINUTES):

Take YES to 5 and walk with purpose and poise for the next 5 minutes. Your effort should feel *potent* but not the least bit stressful. It should feel *steady* but not at all strenuous.

Note to Your Inner Coach

Trust Yourself

When you train for life, you're not just training your muscles — you're training your Inner Coach! That means paying attention to the signals your body is giving you and making changes wherever necessary. Safety comes first, always. If you find it difficult to walk and safely perform the upper-body exercises, then slow your pace down. If that doesn't help, stop and do the upper-body intervals without walking. It may take a little longer, but you'll get the benefits of both safely.

Similarly, if you discover that one exercise feels really uncomfortable, unnatural, or painful for your body, don't do it. You're putting yourself at greater risk of an injury.

I trust that you are giving me your best efforts and that your intention is to improve, to follow my instructions, and to get a great WorkOut. You know when something feels wrong. Part of taking good care of yourself is learning not to extend beyond your responsible limits for yourself or for anyone — including me.

STEP 6 (41–43 MINUTES):
Dial down YES to 4 for the next 3 minutes. Use this subtle reduction from physical intensity to go inside; there's plenty to think about! Keep walking steadily as you repeat your WorkIn: recovery is a necessity, not a luxury.

STEP 7 (44–48 MINUTES):
Over the next 5 minutes, gradually decrease YES from 4 to 3 to 2 and finally to 1.

You'll feel your breathing return to its most relaxed state pretty quickly. Feel how warm, worked out, and relaxed you are right now. Now turn your attention inward; after all, that's what the recovery days are for. The point of Training for Life isn't just to survive — it's to *thrive,* and recovery is an integral part of that process. I want

> ### TRAINING TIP
>
> This may seem like another contradiction in terms, but try to keep your muscles relaxed as you do these exercises. Like a firm massage, these exercises should feel powerfully deep, but *good.* You must — and will — learn to recognize the difference between muscular effort and pain, and you should never sacrifice your well-being for an exercise.
>
> Notice when your neck hurts, your shoulders tense up, or your back becomes sore, and make adjustments accordingly: adjust your arm and shoulder position, pull in your abdominal muscles to protect your lower back, and take a break if necessary. An overall mind-body check-in can help you to "reset" your posture and form.

you to feel good throughout the day and look forward to a lovely evening, no matter what's in store for you when you get home — that's much easier when you know you give yourself the time to rejuvenate. When you give yourself the time you need to rest on a regular basis, you'll improve your strength, your endurance, and your attitude.

You've seen how it works during your WorkOuts, and I guarantee that regularly building these recovery periods into your days will make them even more enjoyable, too. For these last 5 minutes, turn your attention to how and where you will begin building these recovery periods into your life.

Stretch

Find a stable wall (a tree or a fence will work fine) that you can use to stretch out your upper and lower body.

CALF STRETCH

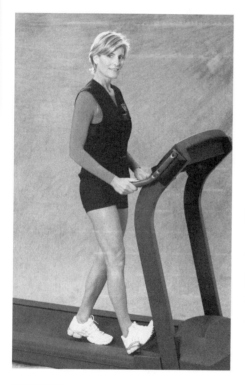

Stand very close to the stable structure and put one foot against it so that your toes and the ball of your foot are pushing against it while your heel remains on the ground. Balance yourself with the foot behind you. Lean toward the structure, pressing the heel of your front foot down while reaching the toes up so you can feel the stretch in your calf. Hold for 10 seconds. If you want a more intense stretch, move even closer to the wall. You may feel this all the way up the back of your leg into your hamstring; that's great! Hold for another 10 seconds and switch legs. Do 2 sets of 2 repetitions, held for 10 seconds on each side.

KNEELING QUAD STRETCH

Note: This may be uncomfortable (or impossible) for you; if so, do the next quad stretch instead.

Sit down on your bent knees, with your rear end and body weight resting on your heels and calves. Lift, as you do while walking, through the top of your head so that your back is straight and you're sitting lightly on your legs as your quadriceps muscles release. If this is comfortable, and you could use a bit more stretch, lean back slightly, using your hands for support behind you. Imagine pushing energy forward, through the kneecaps, to lengthen the quads. Hold for 10 seconds, sit up, release, and repeat.

STANDING QUAD STRETCH

Turn around so your back is toward the wall. Bend your leg behind you and grab the foot of the leg you've bent behind you.

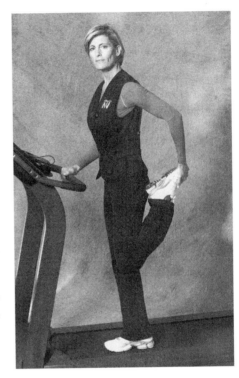

If you're very flexible and want more intensity, back up toward the wall and pull up slightly on your foot while gently pressing your bent knee toward the ground.

If this is difficult, rest the top of your foot on a chair or a bench behind you instead. For a deeper stretch press the top of your foot against your support.

Whichever version you choose, hold it for a count of 10, giving your muscles ample time to release, lengthen, and relax.

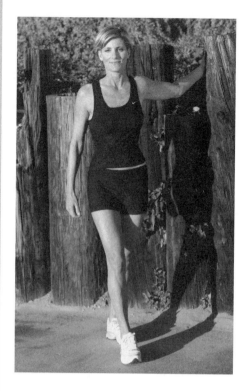

CHEST STRETCH

Move an arm's length away from the wall and stand with your side to it. Place your palm on the wall at shoulder height, with your fingers facing backward, and gently turn your upper body so that you feel a stretch in your shoulder, arms, and chest. Hold for 10 seconds, release, and do the same on your other side. Do 2 sets on each side. Change the placement of your hand (above and below shoulder height); feel how many different areas in your chest and arms this stretch can reach.

CHAPTER 12

Training Day Four: Strength

Let Go of the Results

"Wise are those who learn that the bottom line doesn't always have to be their top priority."

—WILLIAM WARD, SCHOLAR, AUTHOR, AND PASTOR

Part of true strength is having, in the words of the famous prayer, the serenity to accept the things you cannot change, the courage to change the things you can, and the wisdom to know the difference.

Though you are entirely responsible for the quality and consistency of your efforts, you cannot control, or predict, the results. There is just no way to know how fast you will lose the weight, what your butt will look like after seven days, how a new butt will affect your romantic life, or how your friends and family will react to the new you. In order to succeed and achieve total fitness, you will have to **let go of the results and your expectations about them.**

That's hard. We're a result-oriented culture — so much so that we let our results, both the good and the bad, dictate how we feel about ourselves. But it's a seriously flawed system. Don't you see how dangerous it is to prop up your self-esteem on the one thing *you don't control?* When our results don't live up to our expectations (and they rarely do, since our expectations are usually quite unrealistic), we lose interest, sabotage ourselves, and quit.

Life isn't predictable, and neither is weight loss. No one can predict the future — although predicting the future is exactly what most diets claim to do when they tell you that you'll lose X pounds in Y amount of time. Even when you're doing everything right, you will inevitably go through periods when your body resists change and your progress slows down or stops for a bit. If your willingness to stay on the road is conditional on the expectation of certain results, then it won't be long before you begin to backslide. On the other hand, if you're concerned only with your actions, you're always successful. Results will come, in the same way that the kettle will boil; but the more you focus on those results, the slower it will seem.

I need you now to recognize the importance and the magnitude of your *efforts*, not the end product. When you shift your focus from your results, which you don't control, to your efforts, which you *do*, you'll be free to do your WorkOuts in a pure, uncomplicated, and unconditional way.

Put your energy into your *efforts*, not the results, and you will always be triumphant.

So today stay in the present, do your work as suggested, and let go of your expectations. Concentrate on your intention to do the best you can: your efforts will reflect your intention, and your unexpectedly fabulous results will reflect your effort. I guarantee you that if you give each WorkOut a pure and dedicated effort, you will always feel great about *you* at the end. That's more important than anything else. For the best rewards of all, give your best efforts in every training session.

WorkIn: My best effort is my greatest reward. I know that the results are not up to me, so I will stay focused on what I *do* control: my efforts. I will surely *get* more when I *give* more.

Training for Life Meals

Breakfast: a three-egg-white omelet with mushroom, tomato, spinach, and onion (or any similar mix of vegetables) and an orange.

Lunch: one or two cups of fresh green salad with two to four ounces of canned tuna or salmon (packed in water) and three to four tablespoons of dressing. One slice whole-grain (wheat free if possible) bread or toast with no butter or one-half cup steamed whole-grain brown or basmati rice.

Dinner: high-protein kebabs. Skewer two kebabs with two chunks of each: tomato, mushroom, onion, and protein (chicken, fish, or tofu). Serve with two cups of green salad or cucumber-and-tomato salad (one-half large or whole small cucumber and one small or one-half large tomato chopped in chunks, sprinkled with dressing, rice wine, or balsamic vinegar).

Snack: ten raw almonds.

Over the course of the day, drink eight 8-ounce glasses of water.

Strength WorkOut

DAY FOUR WALKOUT

STEP 1 (1–5 MINUTES):

Warm-up: For the first 5 minutes, gradually increase Your Effort Scale from 1 to 3. This is a time to position yourself, physically and mentally, for your WalkOut by agreeing to concentrate exclusively on your efforts.

Position your body by bringing focus to your posture, remembering to stride naturally and lightly, and engaging your core (pull the WalkVest belt tight if you're wearing one). Relax your upper body and shake or roll out any tension that you feel in your arms, hands, shoulders, neck, etc. Position yourself mentally for the WorkOut by recognizing that your mind is as much a part of the training as is your body. It's your mind that controls your awareness, intentions, and actions — your efforts, in other words.

STEP 2 (6–15 MINUTES):

We will spend the next segment of the workout gradually increasing your effort scale.

Start by increasing YES to 4 and walk at this level for the next 5 minutes. Then increase to YES 5 for another 5 minutes. This mid-range level of cardio intensity should feel powerful, but it should not be too strenuous for you to maintain comfortably for the full 5 minutes. Concentrate on keeping your breathing steady and regular, just as your pace is steady and regular.

> ### TRAINING TIP
>
> It's completely normal for your breathing to become a little stressed as you increase the intensity of the work you're doing; it will settle in a few moments. The fitter you become, the more quickly this will happen.

STEP 3 (16–20 MINUTES):
Upper-Body WorkOut: Open Heart

Maintain your pace, keeping Your Effort Scale at 5.

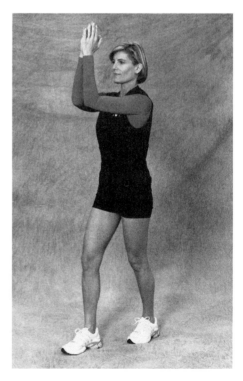

Bring your arms to field-goal position: arms bent at a right angle, fingertips to the sky. Keep your forearms perpendicular to the ground and your upper arms parallel to it as you bring your elbows together in front of you and touch them together, if you can. Hold for 2 counts.

DAY FOUR STRENGTH WORKOUT

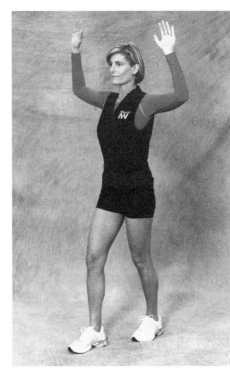

Then, keeping the movement fluid, open the elbows, bringing them as far back behind you as you can, and hold for another count of 2. Here you should feel a stretch as you try to squeeze your shoulder blades together.

As you open your arms, I'd like you to imagine that you are not just elongating the muscles in your chest but literally *opening your heart.* Done regularly, this exercise will allow you greater flexibility, openness, and receptivity in your body, heart, and mind.

Practice 4 sets of open heart over the course of the next 5 minutes, with Level I doing 8 repetitions and Level II doing 15 repetitions each. After each set, release your arms by your sides and keep walking at YES 5. When you've finished your sets, see if you can keep the sensation of feeling open in your heart.

STEP 4 (21–28 MINUTES):

Increase YES to 6 for 4 minutes by increasing your walking speed and incline.

Engage your upper body by adding a subtle pumping action to the movement of your arms. You'll feel the increase in intensity immediately, and your breathing will get deeper as the work requires more effort, but the movement of your arms should also be just what you need to meet the new energy requirement of YES 6.

Intensify YES one more time to 7 and stay here for a powerful 4-minute interval. Focus on the task immediately at hand, doing each interval as it comes, without thinking about the results — they will surely reflect your efforts.

Note to Your Inner Coach

Every Day Is Different

Letting go of the results is not only an effective way to train; it's a compassionate way to train, too.

You're not a machine. Our minds and bodies interact in complex ways, so things may feel different from one day to the next. Yesterday's WorkOut might have felt great, today's not so hot. The beauty of a system like YES is that it can accommodate all your changes. A 5 on Your Effort Scale may take the form of a faster pace on a day when you feel rested and strong and a slower one on a day when you do not — but it will always feel moderate and powerful, according to your particular ability on any given day. As long as you're putting in the amount of effort I've requested, feel proud and accomplished; you're going to get a really effective WorkOut.

Unfortunately we're all so goal-oriented that when we feel "off," our inner voice starts in with the self-doubt and criticism: "I can't do this. This isn't working. I quit." With no wiggle room and no compassion, no wonder it's so hard to succeed.

If — or should I say when? — you hear that voice, simply allow these thoughts to float out of your mind. We are not getting on or off the diet-go-round anymore, so there's no reason to listen or fight with those thoughts; they're the calling cards of your old friend "sabotage," and there's no place for them in Training for Life. Crowd them out by bringing your focus back to your efforts, because when you contribute an honest effort — no matter what that effort looks like today — you're doing what you need to do to get the results you want.

STEP 5 (29–31 MINUTES):

Increase YES to 8 for 2 minutes. Swing your arms to increase your pace and the level of intensity. Stay here for 2 minutes; focus on nothing but the effort you are contributing, then increase YES to 9 for 1 minute. I know you can do this.

Note to Your Inner Coach

Enjoy the Ride

Asking you to let go of the results is just another way to get you to enjoy the journey more. Result-oriented conditioning has taken all the fun out of "getting there," and workouts are no exception: we rob ourselves of a pleasurable experience by focusing exclusively on the end results. My goal is to have you enjoy your life to the fullest extent possible — embracing every step in the journey, not just reaching the destination.

Think about dancing. You dance because you want to. Nobody dances to get to the other side of the dance floor; we do it purely out of joy. Today dance through your WorkOut, reveling in the way it feels to have your muscles moving, your blood pumping, and some time spent just taking care of you. Of course your WorkOuts will have a great impact on your body, but let me worry about that — today come to your WorkOut just for fun.

Remember that you don't control your results, so don't let them control you.

STEP 6 (32–36 MINUTES):

Return YES to 5 and feel the relief as you catch your breath. Stay present, focused, and aware of how you feel as you steadily recover, walking softly for the next 5 minutes.

Take this time to do a mind-body check-in (see page 74), as if you were pressing a reset button to bring your breathing, posture, and stride back into focus and proper form.

STEP 7 (37–46 MINUTES):

In this sequence the work will become increasingly intense, but for shorter periods of time. Know that moving your heart rate up and down and working at various levels of intensity for various amounts of

> **TRAINING TIP**
>
> It's easy to get sloppy when you're working at faster speeds and higher levels of intensity, but it's critical to make sure that you don't ever sacrifice form for speed. Heighten your awareness as well as your physical power, and you can have both.

time throughout the WalkOut will dramatically increase your cardio fitness as well as contribute greatly to rapid weight loss.

Repeat your WorkIn — my best effort is my greatest reward — as you:

- Dial up the volume on YES to 6 for 4 minutes.
- Go to 7 for 3 minutes.
- Increase to 8 for 2 minutes.
- And finally, give me 1 minute at 9.

STEP 8

This is a time for you and your Inner Coach to consider carefully how you feel. You may be able to keep going, and you may be right where you should be. Remember that while stepping out of your comfort zone is a good thing, being reckless is not. Your responsibly powerful and honest efforts will reap you the greatest rewards.

Level I (47–51 minutes):
Proceed to R&R box opposite.

Level II (47–51 minutes):
Ahhh, recovery. Reduce your pace to 5, and you'll feel your breathing ease. Focus on recovering whatever you've lost: your breath, your poise — and the strength of your convictions, if need be.

STEP 9
Level II (52–61 minutes):
Just as you did before, repeat your WorkIn, focus on your efforts, and:

- Dial up the volume on YES to 6 for 4 minutes.
- Go to 7 for 3 minutes.
- Increase to 8 for 2 minutes.
- Finally, give me 1 minute at 9.

Be very aware of each level as you climb one step at a time toward the very top of Your Effort Scale.

STEP 10
Level II (62–64 minutes):

Walk for 3 minutes with YES at 7 and a truly joyous attitude: you're almost home.

STEP 11
Level II (65–69 minutes):

Gorgeous job. Go to the Rest and Reflect box below for your cooldown.

REST AND REFLECT

The Big Picture

Dial YES back *gradually* over the next 5 minutes all the way to 1, taking ample time to return to easy breathing, and allow your body to relax and fully recover. As you walk, consider how you can balance this new skill of focusing on your efforts while still keeping an eye on the big picture.

I know that you've spent the last hour coaching yourself to focus exclusively on your efforts — it's an important practice and a good lesson to take with you. Naturally in life you'll need to keep a bigger-picture view so you know what's coming up and what you'll need to master the tasks of the day. At the same time you don't want to overwhelm yourself by focusing exclusively on the big picture, because then you'll never be able to give your finest effort to what's right in front of you.

Sometimes it's a fine line. Spend too much time on one project at work, and the other ones suffer; not enough, and the end result won't make you proud. Spend too much money on a vacation, and you'll spend the rest of the year haunted by your financial imprudence, but the act of denying yourself a much-needed rest can be even more detrimental to your self-confidence and spirit. Soon you'll naturally be doing your own coaching, as part of taking better care of yourself. As with everything else, the key is balance, and it is that balance that this training will help you to achieve — forever. For now I'll manage the big picture in your WorkOuts so that you can focus on giving me a glorious effort every time.

Stretch, Strengthen, and Tone (approximately 10 minutes)

TRICEPS DIPS (ARMS)

I love this exercise because you can do it anywhere, and it very effectively isolates the muscles that help reel in the dreaded underarm jiggle.

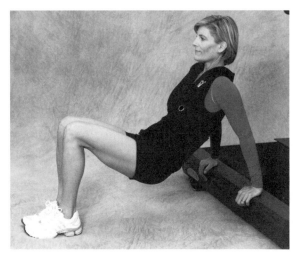

Sit at the edge of a sturdy chair or bench (the second step of a staircase will do as well — anything with a slight elevation). Place your hands on the seat of the bench, on either side of your hips, with your fingers curled around the front edge. Bend your legs so that your heels make contact with the ground and your toes point up toward the ceiling and shift your rear end forward so that it clears the edge of the bench.

Keep your elbows pointed straight back as you bend them to a 90-degree angle and slowly lower your rear end toward the floor. Just as slowly, straighten them again. Repeat.

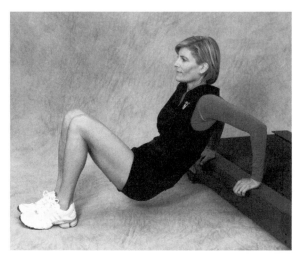

If you need more of a challenge, you can do this exercise with your legs fully extended. If you can successfully do 4 sets with legs bent, I recommend that you try to replace at least 1 bent-leg set with a straight-leg set, gradually working your way to doing all 4 with straight legs.

Level I:

2 sets, 6 repetitions in each set.

Level II:

3 sets, 10 repetitions in each set.

LEG LIFTS (HIPS, THIGHS)

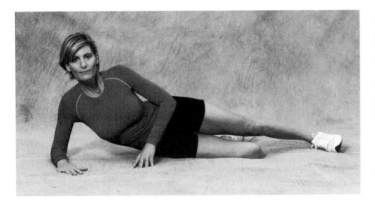

Lie on one side. You can prop yourself on your elbow or put your head on your arm on the ground; the most important thing is that your body is straight, so that your ankle is in a straight line with your knee, hip, and shoulder. Bend the bottom leg to 90

degrees for stability, keeping your leg straight, and your foot lightly flexed, with your toes pointed back toward your face. Raise your leg three inches from the ground. From this position, using a slow and controlled motion, lift your straight leg to the height of your shoulder and

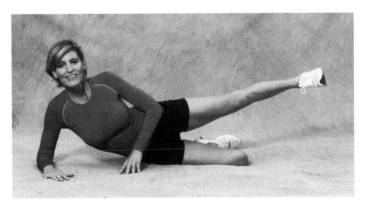

then slowly return it to the starting position, three inches off the ground. Don't lower your upper leg onto your lower leg between counts.

Level I:

2 sets on each side, 10 reps in each set.

Level II:

2 sets on each side, 20 reps in each set.

CRUNCHES (SEE PAGE 83)

Level I:

3 sets of 8.

Level II:

3 sets of 12.

Have a great day — let go of the results and enjoy the process.

CHAPTER 13

Training Day Five: Endurance

Hunger

Hunger is defined as a great need or desire for *something* — not just for food.

Most of us have enormous appetites, but often it's not really food that we desire. Instead we are hungry for love, comfort, success, recognition, validation, or respect. What we hunger for is that our lives be different, *better* than they are now. But we eat over those feelings, using food as a drug, a way to numb ourselves so that we can't feel our loneliness, lack, self-loathing, or anger.

Can you now see why all this eating — and overeating — doesn't actually satisfy you?

There's a better way, a way to put your enormous hunger to good use and make eating a more responsible and pleasurable activity. It's time to see your hunger as a resource, a productive and vital tool, and to use this powerful drive to transform your body and your life. After all, the feelings behind the hunger — dissatisfaction, ambition, restlessness — can also produce in us a very healthy yearning for change. Your hunger means that you are a striver and that you want more from life: more joy, more money, more love, more fun, more sex, more choices, more freedom, and more success. In TFL we'll harness that energy to benefit you.

So today when you feel hungry, don't eat over it or do anything else to mask it — just let it be. In fact, see if you can even get closer to it — notice where you feel it in your body and what it feels like. See how long you feel it for and how long it lasts if you don't eat anything right away. Now you have the opportunity to find out just what it is that you're hungry for. Write it down; after all, the first step to true satisfaction is knowing what you really want! Getting in touch with the feelings behind your hunger is an important part of your growth and success; the other option, of course, is to go back and forth to the refrigerator, packing on the extra pounds, and never getting any kind of meaningful satisfaction.

Allow the hunger today, even embrace it: I guarantee that you will be enriched by what you learn when you don't eat to silence it.

WorkIn: My hunger is my desire to succeed. I will no longer silence my ambitions with food.

Training for Life Meals

Breakfast: one cup puffed rice or Kashi cereal (no sugar added) with nonfat milk and one-half cup of berries.

Lunch: bunless chicken, turkey, soy, or veggie burger topped with lettuce and tomato, one-half tablespoon ketchup and/or mustard, with one cup of vegetable soup or steamed veggies.

Dinner: salad. To two cups of fresh salad, add one-quarter cup of prepared garbanzo, soy, or kidney beans (or mix of all three), one-quarter cup cooked peas, and one-quarter avocado. Sprinkle with two to four tablespoons of your favorite dressing. Eat with one slice of whole-grain bread or toast (wheat free preferably) or one-half cup whole-grain rice, quinoa, or millet.

Snacks: ten almonds; one mango or papaya.

Over the course of the day, drink eight 8-ounce glasses of water.

Endurance WorkOut

DAY FIVE WALKOUT

STEP 1 (1–5 MINUTES):

Warm-up: Walk easily at YES 1 to warm up your body, gradually increasing your pace to YES 3. Lift out of the crown of your head and stand erect, so you are walking tall and stepping lightly.

STEP 2 (6–20 MINUTES):

Over the next 15 minutes, you'll walk at increasingly intense 5-minute intervals. As the intensity escalates, so will your heart rate and the number of calories you burn with every step! Don't forget to consciously notice and manage your breathing, keeping it steady and even.

Engage your abs and reach the top of your head toward the sky.

- Speed your pace to YES 4 and stay there for 5 minutes.
- Increase to YES 5 for 5 minutes.
- Go to YES 6 for 5 minutes.

Note to Your Inner Coach

Put Pride in Your Stride

As you know, your actions reflect your thoughts, beliefs, and feelings. You can (and must) *think* your way into behaving differently. That is why our training, which is meant to improve your life, not just your physical appearance, includes conditioning for the mind as well as the physical body.

It works the other way around, too. You can (and must) *act* your way into new thinking. These actions may be as simple as walking tall, as though you have confidence and poise to spare, on a day when you don't feel like you've got any at all. Other techniques include refraining from eating certain foods for a while, which changes your behavior and reconditions your feelings in order to weaken a previously unmanageable craving.

It's in the name of "acting your way to better thinking" that I am asking you to do things differently, right off the bat, even *before* you believe, understand, or fully embrace what we are doing in Training for Life. These behavioral changes are not the complete picture — as you know, I don't think *any* permanent change can take place unless you've changed your mind as well. But they are still a very important part of the reconditioning process, especially at the beginning.

Ultimately the best and most efficient way to create permanent change is to condition ourselves inside and out, *acting* and *thinking* together. But faking it until you get there can help you make it through a rough patch, especially in the early days, until your Inner Coach takes over.

So walk with pride in your stride, no matter how you feel today.

STEP 3 (21–25 MINUTES):

Dial YES back slowly, from 6 to 4.

Don't let go of your training senses during recovery. Remember that recovery is an important part of your training, *not a break from it.*

Repeat your WorkIn — my hunger is my desire to succeed. Use this time to refuel and regroup.

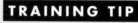

TRAINING TIP

Be sure to drink water during your recovery periods so you stay hydrated.

STEP 4 (26–35 MINUTES):
Open Heart:

It's time to tap into your hunger; we're going to escalate the intensity again by doing some strength and toning work for your upper body.

Increase YES from 4 to 5. You'll stay at this intensity for 10 minutes while adding 4 sets of 10 (for Level I) and 4 sets of 20 (for Level II) open hearts (see page 108) for the upper body, with 30 seconds of recovery in between sets. Your Effort Scale may increase as you add these exercises; maintain YES 5 by reducing your pace if necessary. Maintain your walking posture and the integrity of your stride whenever you add upper-body work.

STEP 5 (36–45 MINUTES):

Walk at YES 6, the highest level of your Moderate Zone, for 5 minutes. Then move to the beginning of your Power Zone, YES 7 for 5 minutes, and feel yourself hungry to succeed.

STEP 6 (46–50 MINUTES):

Turn *down* YES to 4 and recover while still walking tall. Stay focused as you feel your breathing get easier; this is the perfect time for a mind-body check-in. Find your poise, your posture, and your breath.

Note to Your Inner Coach

You don't lack for anything, and you don't need to fear being left "without." Certain behavioral changes can help you send that message, to the universe and to yourself. Here are some of the things that I practice:

First of all, whether in a restaurant or at home, I look at the portion of food on my plate and compare it to what I know about the size of my stomach: that it's the size of a potato! Yours is, too — so what are we doing with steaks too big to fit on a dinner plate and bathtub-size salads? We're stretching our poor stomachs beyond what they can comfortably contain — and making ourselves fat in the process. Save the extra portion for tomorrow and feel good about "enough" as opposed to "too much."

Another thing: I don't eat other people's food. I don't sneak the rest of my son's mac 'n' cheese when I'm cleaning up after dinner or finish my daughter's entrée when she's full. Their food is theirs and mine is mine, and that's the way it should be.

Finally, I leave a small amount of food on the plate every time I eat. I feel that this sends a little message that I am not afraid of being hungry and that I have *more than I need.* I was conditioned, as many of you were, to clean my plate: "There's no dessert if you don't finish your meal" and "There are starving children who'd do anything to have that dinner." But the truth is that overeating doesn't help those children. I have a responsibility to take care of myself, and only when I do that can I take good care of others.

If I have one goal with this program, it's to give you the tools to take better care of yourself and the intrinsic desire to use them. When you realize that feelings can't hurt you, you won't feel the need to silence them with food. And you won't panic when your stomach feels empty (or full, for that matter) because you'll understand there will always be enough of what you really need and that you will always be nourished, body and soul.

STEP 7 (51–62 MINUTES):
Increase YES to 5, then to 6, then to 7, and WalkOut for 4 minutes at each level.

STEP 8
Level I (63–67 minutes):

Great work. Go to the box below for some R&R.

Level II (63–65 minutes):

Take 3 minutes at YES 4 to recover your breathing and your comfortable stride.

STEP 9
Level II (66–77 minutes):

Escalate YES in 4-minute intervals, YES 5 to YES 6 to YES 7. Keep the pride in your stride as you head into the homestretch.

STEP 10
Level II (78–80 minutes):

Drop YES to 6 and walk for 3 minutes. Remember, your hunger will keep you strong, focused on your goals, and steady on the road, so embrace it.

STEP 11
Level II (81–85 minutes):

Great work — another one well done. Go to the R&R box below.

REST AND REFLECT

Little by little, over the next 5 minutes, take yourself all the way back to YES 1. Walk with a keen awareness of your achievement today and congratulate yourself on a WalkOut well done.

Here's something to digest as you walk. Our automatic reaction when we feel the physical sensation of hunger is to feed it, squelch it, eliminate it — and any feelings that come with it. I wonder why we are so afraid to be physically hungry? Do we think we'll starve, with a convenience store on every corner? Is it a holdover from our ancestors who didn't have such reliable access to food?

DAY FIVE ENDURANCE WORKOUT

I'm concerned that it's the feeling of *desire* that we're eliminating. Maybe we were taught at a young age that having strong passions and desires isn't appropriate or seemly. Maybe our desires frustrate or frighten us because we've never been given the tools to achieve them. Maybe feeling *anything* makes us uncomfortable. But our desires are what drive us to succeed. Whatever the motivation, it's time to let go of the panic and fear we feel around our hungers so we can get some real nourishment and satisfaction.

You *are* enough, you have enough, and you always will.

The work you're doing as part of Training for Life will help fortify your inner strength — the sense of trust and confidence that you feel in yourself — so that you can turn your attitude about hunger and desire around. Knowing that you are capable and believing in yourself are first steps toward knowing that your desires are valid and attainable. This is a terrific antidote to the fears that our hungers call up in us.

Stretch and Abs (approximately 10 minutes)

If you are wearing a WalkVest, remove it for this portion of the WorkOut.

SNOW ANGEL

Lie flat on your back with your arms and legs spread as wide as they can possibly go. Stretch, open, and reach away from your body, as if you were being gently pulled by your fingers and toes. Hold the stretch for 10 seconds and then *release*. Stay in this relaxed mode for 20 seconds, letting your body become super heavy and loose as it sinks into the ground. Repeat the sequence, reaching for 10 seconds and relaxing for 20, 2 more times.

CRUNCHES (SEE PAGE 83)

Level I:

3 sets of 8.

Level II:

3 sets of 10.

Recover with a Snow Angel.

CRUNCHES (SEE PAGE 83)

Level I:

3 sets of 8.

Level II:

3 sets of 10.

Recover with another Snow Angel — notice how good it feels to stretch the muscles you've just worked!

CHILD'S POSE

Sit on your heels (or as close as possible), round your back, and try to tuck your forehead into your knees so that the top of your head touches the floor. Fold your arms in front of you and make a pillow for your forehead, stretch your arms out in front of you for a back stretch, or bring them to rest by your sides. Hold the pose for 20 to 30 seconds. Feel the warmth of your breath as it cleanses, relaxes, and revitalizes your body.

Feel and absorb all the changes in your body that have taken place over the course of your WorkOut. Slowly get to your feet and take a deep breath as you stretch your arms above your head for one tranquility pose.

Have the day you hunger for!

Training Day Six: Endurance

Choosing "Right" Instead of "Right Now"

"Knowing is not enough; we must apply. Willing is not enough; we must do."

— GOETHE

Every day we're faced with a series of choices. What you're going to work on today is how you can make the *right* choice, instead of the one that feels good right now.

The difference between "right" and "right now" is the difference between a quick fix and a useful solution, the difference between something that's going to make you *feel* better in the moment and something that's actually going to make *you* better.

Here's my wish for you: that all the decisions you make from here on be made with awareness, an honest recognition of all consequences. With awareness you **create the space between thought and action** so that you can recognize the difference between "right" and "right now" choices and give yourself the opportunity to choose more wisely.

Training for Life is designed to help you hone that awareness. Let's say that you come home from work late, exhausted after an exceptionally grueling day. Instead of mindlessly devouring take-out Chinese and watching two hours of TV, use what little energy you have left to make a healthful food choice — one that's just as simple and easy as a take-out dinner — and then get right into bed; I don't care what time it is. Turn the phone off, put up the "do not disturb" sign, ask someone else to do what needs to get done, and get as much sleep as you possibly can. You will feel *truly* revived in the morning — rather than hung over from a greasy fix and a late night of TV.

Here's another one: It's 4:30 in the afternoon, and the office vending machine beckons. All you need to get through your daily mid-afternoon energy lull is a little yellow pack of M&Ms or one of those frothy coffee confections, right? Wrong — that's "right now" thinking. Sugar, fat, and caffeine are no good for you, even at the best of times, and they have an even more adverse effect on you when you're mentally and physically vulnerable. Your body is definitely telling you that you need something, but you can choose a quick fix that will give you immediate gratification (and unpleasant ramifications later) or you can choose better and make an investment in the rest of your afternoon.

Awareness gives you space between thought and action. Before you hit the coffee bar or the vending machine, you can ask yourself, "Is it food that I need, or would a five-minute walk clear my head?" And if a walk doesn't suffice, then choose a snack that won't make your blood sugar skyrocket and then crash, ultimately making you hungrier (not to mention fat!). When you choose an apple over a candy bar; a cup of soup over a cookie; or a few slices of turkey, a small can of tuna, or half a dozen almonds over a frozen yogurt, you're choosing "right" over "right now."

When your choices are made with awareness and thoughtfulness instead of through habit or reaction, you can make more of them healthy. Still, I know that you're going to make the "right now" decision every once in a while. That's fine — those are a part of life, too, and I do want you to live a life that's fun, and full, and free. Being too restrictive can be as bad as being too indulgent, and the line between "right" and "right now" won't always be so clearly defined. But when you live your life consciously, thoughtfully, and with awareness, you can knowingly choose a muffin (every once in a while), and it won't throw you into a tailspin or send you back to binging and dieting.

Learning to make the "right" choices may take some self-discipline in the beginning. As author and publisher Elbert Hubbard put it in the nineteenth century, you'll need "the ability to make yourself do what you should do, when you should do it, whether you feel like it or not" — but *only* in the beginning. Why? Because Training for Life is conditioning your mind to *want* to take better care of your body, so that soon your choices will automatically and instinctively be healthier.

I don't want you to have to white-knuckle your life, with self-discipline being the only thing standing between the "new you" and the way you were. As you train for life, you will quickly appreciate how good it feels to be strong, lean, balanced, and energetic as opposed to overweight, lethargic, reactive, tired, defeated, and guilty. But an appreciation for the good life clearly isn't enough — or it would have stuck at least one of the other times you'd begun a new regimen and lost weight. Training your mind as well as your body will ensure that your decision to exercise regularly and eat healthily will become *who you are,* not just what you do. Changing the way you think, as well as the way you behave, will make it easy to choose the things that support feeling and looking good.

WorkIn: I'd rather *be* better than feel better temporarily. I will give myself what I really need when I really need it. Choosing *right* means that I consider my choices carefully.

Training for Life Meals

Breakfast: one slice whole-grain bread (sugar free and wheat free, if possible), topped with one-quarter cup of low-fat or nonfat cottage cheese and berries (optional).

Lunch: two cups of steamed or lightly sautéed veggies with one-half cup whole-grain brown rice.

Dinner: chili. Layer or mix together two cups of steamed vegetables chopped in small chunks; four ounces (or one-half cup) cooked, chopped, or ground chicken, turkey, or soy protein; and one-quarter cup of sugar-free tomato sauce. Serve with cucumber-and-tomato salad.

Snacks: ten almonds, one grapefruit.

Over the course of the day, drink eight 8-ounce glasses of water.

Endurance WorkOut

DAY SIX WALKOUT

STEP 1 (1–5 MINUTES):

Warm-up: Walk easily, going from the very bottom of Your Effort Scale to 3 in the first 5 minutes of your WalkOut.

Take your time and indulge yourself in this warmup period. Feel your body waking up. Roll your shoulders and rub your hands together quickly to generate some heat as you pick up your pace a little bit to do the same for the rest of your body.

STEP 2 (6–25 MINUTES):

Walk with increasing intensity, in 4 increments of 5 minutes each. I love these long endurance interval sequences because they give you the opportunity to fully experience each level — physically and mentally — of the endurance conditioning.

Increase YES to 4 and walk with relaxed shoulders and arms, and a light stride, for 5 minutes. Then go to YES 5 for 5 minutes, increasing your intensity just a bit. Add arm movement for momentum as you go to YES 6 for 5 more minutes. Then, bravely and without hesitation, walk powerfully at YES 7 for 5 minutes more.

STEP 3 (26–30 MINUTES):

Dial down YES to 4 for a nice, steady recovery interval.

At YES 4 you still must maintain a vital and energetic stride, but because you've come from YES 7, it should feel easy, relaxing, and a great relief. Stay focused on your posture: keep your abs engaged and your arms relaxed as you walk tall. Remember, a responsible amount of recovery in each day is the "right" choice.

STEP 4 (31–45 MINUTES):

Repeat Step 2. This time you'll do 3 intervals of 5 minutes each, going from YES 5 to 6 to 7.

Note to Your Inner Coach

Learn to Endure

A big part of choosing "right" over "right now" is having the ability to stay with something, even when it's not what you want at that moment.

Going *all the way* with your WorkOut, mentally and physically, can be uncomfortable, especially when I ask you for more (and more and more) intensity. It's natural for you to react to that discomfort by thinking about stopping; you may even dress up your excuse by remembering something absolutely essential that needs to be done right away. But here again you have a choice. Choosing to stop is the "right now" choice; sticking with it is the *right* one.

Endurance training will help move you past the roadblocks that you (consciously or unconsciously) have set up, barriers that keep you right where you are, even though you say that you want to change. Endurance training teaches you to feel your discomfort while still moving closer to your goals. It helps you to make the *right* choices, instead of the *right now* ones, so that your life continues to change for the better, even on the days when your heart isn't in it.

By all means acknowledge your feelings — just know that you'll feel better if you don't act on them. Recognize discomfort, but don't move off the level of intensity that I have prescribed until the time is up. Stay with the endurance conditioning, and you will keep moving in a positive direction.

Let's face it — you have places to go, goals to meet, and a better life to live. Let's get there sooner rather than later.

STEP 5 (46–50 MINUTES):

Dial YES to 5 and walk your heart rate down. Again you'll be recovering in your Moderate Zone, but this time at YES 5. The *right* choice for you right now is to stay very present in your WalkOut. Relax in your stride and enjoy the ride as you repeat your WorkIn for the day: I'd rather *be* better than feel better temporarily.

STEP 6 (51–60 MINUTES):

You'll do 2 intervals of 5 minutes each.

Increase YES to 6 for 5 minutes and then again to 7 for 5 minutes. Ease right into your Power Zone and give me — give *yourself* — the purest effort you can muster.

STEP 7 (61–65 MINUTES):

Dial YES back to 6 and walk for 5 minutes. This is just the slightest reduction in intensity, but you should feel it. Your breathing gets easier as your pace gets slightly slower. Stay tuned in to your form and be sure to maintain a clear and conscious awareness of your purpose — to stay steady and strong on the road, to go all the way, and to make the *right* choices more often.

STEP 8
Level I (66–70 minutes):

Excellent work! You can proceed to the R&R box opposite.

Level II (66–70 minutes):

Dial YES up to 7 and walk for 5 minutes. Stay in it and stay strong. Maintain a natural and comfortable stride and don't forget you can use your upper body to help propel your lower body by swinging your arms.

STEP 9
Level II (71–73 minutes):

Go, with everything that you have left, to YES 8 for 2 minutes and YES 9 for 1 minute.

You are almost home — even more reason to focus your energy on sustaining your efforts to the end. Make it a good finish, a worthy finish — a finish you can be proud of.

STEP 10
Level II (74–78 minutes):

Excellent work! Go to the R&R box opposite.

REST AND REFLECT
Reinforce the Positive

Reduce YES slowly, all the way to 1.

As you cool down, here's one last thought. You know that life is a series of choices. Since the life you're living right now is the sum of all the choices you've made up until now, and the choices you make today and tomorrow will determine the life you live in the future, there are lots of good reasons to make the right ones.

Making better choices is something we'd all like to do, but it's hard! If it were easy, we'd all be exactly where we wanted to be. But often our behavior defies logic, and certainly our stated goals: "I *want* to lose weight, I really do. But I can't seem to stop the compulsive nighttime eating. . . ."

There are lots of factors contributing to whether we make the right or wrong choices. Some of them take place at a level so deeply subconscious that we're genuinely ignorant of our motives. That's scary. If we don't even know what the factors are that contribute to the choices we make, how can we change them and reverse their effects? If you don't acknowledge that there's something deeper driving the late-night snacking, how in the world are you going to stop?

The WorkIns you're doing will help to fortify the things we say we *do* want, so that those factors get bigger and stronger in our minds.

Reinforcing the positive weakens the negative.

Affirming the very best of what we want for ourselves gives us the ability to choose healthier, happier, more self-enhancing choices from a place deep inside, one previously inhabited by self-defeating beliefs. It's a self-fulfilling prophecy, as well. The more you make the "right" choices, the more of a foundation you will build to support all of your efforts, today and beyond.

To be sure, it's been a good day already. By showing up and giving me the effort I've asked you for and staying with it, you've demonstrated your ability to choose right instead of right now. Good for you!

Stretch and Abs (approximately 10 minutes)

If you're wearing a WalkVest, remove it.

CRUNCHES
(SEE PAGE 83)

Level I:
3 sets of 8.

Level II:
3 sets of 15.

SINGLE KNEE HUG (SEE PAGE 82)

Hold for 10 to 20 seconds and repeat.

ABCYCLE

Lie on your back and lift your head and shoulders, supporting your upper body with your elbows. Bring your knees into your chest, keeping your lower legs parallel to the ground. As if you were on a bicycle, straighten one leg and then the other, always keeping your feet off the ground.

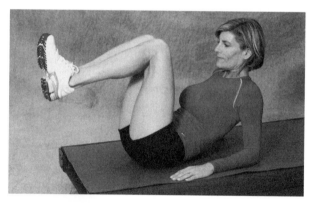

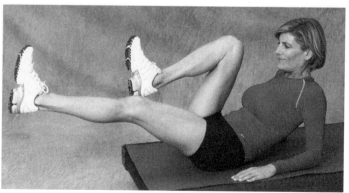

Keep your abdominal muscles contracted and your lower back pressed tightly against the floor. If your lower back hurts, don't fully extend the straightened leg, but keep a slight bend instead.

Level I:

2 sets of 8 on each side.

Level II:

3 sets of 12 on each side.

TOTAL RELEASE

TRAINING TIP

If this exercise strains your lower back, keep your legs closer to your body or sit up a little taller on your elbows.

Lie on your back and relax your body completely for the final few minutes of your WorkOut, letting yourself melt into the ground. Free your body of any leftover tension by melting, mentally and physically, into the floor. Slowly rock your head side to side to release your neck. Then, without moving your head — eyes only! — look up, then down, then side to side. Close your eyes completely now and see if you can *feel* yourself (and enjoy the glory of your accomplishment) more completely.

Stay here for 1 or 2 minutes.

Very slowly rise to your feet and go out to live your day in the right way.

CHAPTER 15

Training Day Seven: Strength

Embrace Resistance

"Adversity causes some men to break; others to break records."

—WILLIAM WARD, SCHOLAR, AUTHOR, AND PASTOR

There's a dual focus to these fourteen days. You're taking in a lot of information, both emotional and practical — a whole new belief system, in fact. You're also learning *to let go* of all the old, self-defeating feelings and beliefs that have trapped you in a life that is less than you deserve. Today you're going to do both at once, as we put a fresh spin on the concept of resistance.

We traditionally think of resistance as a force that works against us. It's something that holds us back: a drag, both literally and figuratively. As a result we look for ways to avoid it. When we have to face it, we brace ourselves against it, fighting it every inch of the way.

Today I'd like you to do something different; I want you to **embrace resistance** instead.

The fact is, resistance is everywhere, and thank goodness for it. Without it we'd literally float away — gravity, after all, is resistance. And we need resistance to strengthen us, physically and mentally. Weight resistance makes our muscles and bones strong, just as an opposing perspective or a challenging conversation can help us arrive at more thoughtful opinions and decisions.

Resistance is the stuff that makes us strong.

It also makes our accomplishments count; without resistance there would be no glory, no victory, no sense of well-earned accomplishment. And resistance gives us perspective — after all, without "hard," there's no "easy."

The bottom line is that resistance is good for us, and there's no question that it's here to stay. And yet we routinely exhaust our mental and physical resources fighting it, avoiding it, or trying to find a way around it. Wouldn't it simply be easier if we learned to embrace it?

Resistance is necessary; struggle is not.

Think about biking into a headwind. You can thrash against the weather angrily, flailing and catching wind so that you arrive at your destination physically and emotionally spent — but I can tell you from experience that no matter how valiant your struggle, the wind won't be affected by *you* at all. You can wait for hours until the headwind passes or take yourself way off course trying to avoid it. That's all just energy squandered and time wasted; some resistance can't be avoided.

Consider this alternative: relax, drop your head, tuck your body into an aerodynamic position, and ride right through the center of it. Embracing the resistance allows us to do our work in the most productive and energy-efficient way, especially since it's not the wind alone that wears us out but the energy we spend fighting it, anticipating it, worrying about it, dragging our heels, and then resenting it every inch of the way. You can preserve your body, your mind, and your energy simply by changing the way you approach resistance. Fighting it only creates more of it, and that doesn't make any sense at all. A more direct approach costs less energy-wise, takes you quickly to where you want to go, and strengthens you in the process.

Resistance will always be a part of our lives, but you can certainly live without *struggle*. So whenever and wherever resistance appears — in your career, on the freeway, in your WorkOuts, in your relationships with others, or in the relationship you have with yourself — apply to it these practical and positive attributes instead of holding on to the idea that it is there to bother or deter you. Recognize resistance for what it is: a natural resource, one that is useful for strengthening both your body and your mind. Understand that embracing it will eliminate the struggle and make your journey much more pleasurable.

WorkIn: Resistance is necessary; struggle is not. Resistance makes me stronger. It is, and always will be, a part of my life.

Training for Life Meals

Breakfast: One grapefruit or papaya and one or two soft-boiled or poached eggs, three tomato slices, and five cucumber slices.

Lunch: one cup or can of soup and two cups of fresh salad (sprinkled with dressing) and one slice whole-grain (wheat free if possible) bread or toast, with one-half cup cottage cheese and ten almonds.

Dinner: four to six ounces grilled or baked salmon or chicken with one-half cup cooked whole-grain rice and two cups salad.

There's no snack today; I don't think it's a good idea to condition you to want one every day. Know that each meal has plenty of food to carry you through.

Over the course of the day, drink eight 8-ounce glasses of water.

Strength WorkOut

DAY SEVEN WALKOUT

STEP 1 (1–5 MINUTES):

Warm-up: Gently, over the next 5 minutes, increase YES from 1 to 3. As you walk, notice the ease with which you are traveling. Memorize the effortless feeling of your erect posture and carriage so that you can tap back into this feeling when you are recovering from work that is more intense.

STEP 2 (6–17 MINUTES):

You'll do three 4-minute intervals, of increasing intensity. Increase YES to 4 for 4 minutes, to 5 for 4 minutes, and to 6 for 4 minutes more.

At each level make a conscious attempt to immerse yourself in the intensity, whether moderate or more powerful. Stay keenly tuned in to your breathing, your posture, and your attitude toward the work.

STEP 3 (18–26 MINUTES):

In this sequence you'll have 3 intervals of 2 minutes each at YES 7, followed by a 1-minute recovery interval in between at YES 5.

Go to YES 7 for 2 minutes. You're in your Power Zone, and you must maintain posture, composure, and awareness throughout, although your breathing will be deep and somewhat stressful. You will use your arms to help propel your legs, and your mind to calm your body, as you adjust to and embrace the intensity.

Then recover at YES 5 for 1 minute. Repeat this sequence 3 times.

Note to Your Inner Coach

Almost every day we find ourselves with piles of work to plow through, miles of traffic to navigate, hills to climb, problems to solve, and more. Wherever and however this work presents itself, help yourself get through it by letting go of your own struggle against it. Use your resources wisely, as you are being trained to do, so that they work *for* and not against you; fighting against resistance always makes the work you have to do harder.

When your effort is required, give it gladly. If you resist, it will persist. Your efforts and energies will go much further if you focus them directly on the task at hand and don't squander them in fruitless protest. Consciously, purposefully, and willingly *embrace the resistance*.

STEP 4 (27–30 MINUTES):

Decrease your efforts to 4 on YES and walk for 4 minutes. Absorb the work that you have just accomplished and refuel for the work ahead.

STEP 5 (31–40 MINUTES):
Walking Lunges

Step off the treadmill (if you're outdoors or in a mall, you can simply slow your pace) for a sequence of walking lunges.

Step out, slightly farther than your normal stride, and bend both knees deeply so that the thigh of your front leg is parallel to the ground. Keep your shoulders relaxed, your chin level to the ground, and your weight evenly distributed. Try not to lean with your hand on your thigh for balance as you lunge.

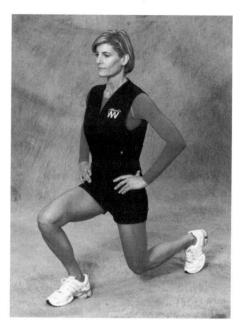

Level I:

3 sets of 8 lunges on each side.

Level II:

5 sets of 10 on each side.

In between sets, walk for approximately 1 minute at YES 5.

STEP 6 (41–46 MINUTES):

Walk at YES 5 for 2 minutes, YES 6 for 2 minutes, and YES 7 for 2 minutes in your Power Zone.

STEP 7 (47–50 MINUTES):

Take 4 minutes at YES 5 to recover your breathing, relax your body, and realign your physical and mental posture.

TRAINING TIP

When you lunge, the knee on your front leg should be positioned *directly* over the ankle. If you're concerned about your form, take a quick peek down: you should always be able to see your toes.

Take your full awareness and attention with you, with every step.

STEP 8 (51–59 MINUTES):

Dial up YES to 6 and walk for 2 minutes, take a 1-minute recovery interval at YES 5, and then dial it up again to YES 7; walk powerfully for 2 minutes there and then recover at YES 5 for 1 minute again.

Finally, dial YES up to 8 and hit it hard for 2 minutes, then recover for 1 minute at YES 5, knowing that you have conquered the resistance in the best way possible, by embracing it.

TRAINING TIP

If you're doing your WalkOuts on a treadmill, crank up the elevation a little higher for added resistance on Strength Training Days.

If you're outside, do your strength training in the hills or on sloping terrain whenever possible.

STEP 9 (60–69 MINUTES):

Walk at YES 5 for 4 minutes, a moderate, but strong pace. Then increase to YES 6 for 3 minutes. Engage your powerful arms to increase YES to 7 for 2 minutes, and then embrace the resistance at YES 8 for a single pure minute.

Note to Your Inner Coach

What's the opposite of going with the flow? Tensing up. The stress we feel in our bodies is the physical manifestation of our resistance to resistance, and it's a good example of how this strategy works against us.

We tend to tense up when faced with a challenging situation. But stress doesn't make us better able to handle the challenges we're presented with, it weakens us by stealing our energy and sound judgment. It makes our muscles knotted and sore and compromises our posture, mental acuity, physical immune systems, and overall sense of well-being.

Challenges are a part of life and help build our mental and physical character. But stress is useless, detrimental, and downright unhealthy — and doesn't have to be a part of our lives at all. Opt out. Refuse to resist resistance, and stress cannot survive. Make it a habit to use the mind-body check-in to recognize and release tension whenever and wherever possible. It's useful during your WorkOuts — or during a long business meeting or a preteen temper tantrum, or when you're stuck in line behind someone counting out five dollars in change.

You'll come up against substantial amounts of resistance during your WalkOuts and in life; you don't need to create any of your own! Practice *not* fighting the hills and headwinds, and you'll see, it's great preparation for moving swiftly through all the obstacles that present themselves in our lives.

STEP 10
Level I (70–74 minutes):
Great job. Move to the R&R box opposite.

Level II (70–72 minutes):
You have 3 minutes to recover at YES 5. Use your time wisely by focusing on reducing your speed, relaxing your breathing, and at the same time maintaining a pace that is moderately strong and steady. Walk tall, scan your body for tension, and relinquish any physical (or mental) stress that you detect.

STEP 11
Level II (73–82 minutes):
Walking Lunge Interval
You have 5 sets of walking lunges to do in the next 10 minutes. Do 10 lunges on each side with a 60-second recovery interval, walking at YES 5 in between. Gather your poise, your power, and your focus, and, as though this were the first exercise of your WalkOut, give me a fresh, vibrant, and powerful set.

TRAINING TIP

You're most likely to get injured when you're tired, which is why it's doubly important to attend to your form as you near the end of your WalkOut.

When you're lunging, pay close attention to foot placement and make sure that your knee never extends past your ankle. Use your core strength to lift up safely from the lunge, rather than relying on just your legs.

STEP 12
Level II (83–87 minutes):
Excellent work. Go to the R&R box below.

REST AND REFLECT

Walk it home with pride, reducing your intensity over the next 5 minutes. Enjoy this final recovery time and your triumph over struggle and resistance.

I'd like to make one thing clear, and it's something you can reflect upon as you cool down. Part of embracing resistance means *noticing* where you struggle in your life, *experiencing* that struggle, *learning* from it, and doing your best to *let it go.* It doesn't mean, however, that you accept difficulty and discomfort passively — there's nothing passive about the life I'm training you for! So although I am encouraging you to embrace resistance, I don't for a minute mean to suggest that you should settle for a relationship, a job, or any situation that's inappropriate, uncomfortable, or less than you deserve. I simply mean that you can use the resistance you feel in those situations to learn about yourself and get to the heart of what's bothering you so that you can deal with it in the most effective way.

For instance, if you wake up every morning filled with dread at the thought of going into your job, don't focus your energy on complaining about your boss or raging against your commute instead of feeling your feelings. Rather, hear what the resistance is telling you: that this job isn't serving you. Use that information to sniff out the root cause of your discontentment — and to change it. Are you resentful that you're not making enough money? Do you need more creative work? What steps can you take to effect these changes?

Embracing resistance means that there is something useful for you and worthy of your attention in it. So as you recover for the last time today, ask yourself if there are areas in your life where you struggle against resistance. If so, given what you know now, could you surrender that struggle and learn from the resistance you feel instead?

Stretch, Strengthen, and Tone (approximately 10 minutes)

If you're wearing a WalkVest, remove it.

TRICEPS DIPS (SEE PAGE 114)

Two sets with legs extended; 2 sets with knees bent.

Note: If the legs-extended version is too stressful on your back or shoulders, do 4 sets with knees bent. If knees bent is not strenuous enough for you, do 4 sets with legs extended.

Level I:

6 repetitions in each set.

Level II:

10 repetitions in each set.

PUSH-UPS (SEE PAGE 79)

Level I:

2 sets of 8.

Level II:

2 sets of 12.

LEG LIFTS (SEE PAGE 115)

2 sets on each side.

Level I:

10 reps in each set.

Level II:

20 reps in each set.

CRUNCHES (SEE PAGE 83)

Level I:
3 sets of 10.

Level II:
3 sets of 15.

SEATED HAMSTRING STRETCH

Sit tall with your legs stretched out in front of you. Imagine, as you do while you're walking, that you're being lifted up through the top of your head and keep your back as straight as possible. Slowly raise your arms up over your head and stretch out of your waist as you lift your fingertips to the sky. Then slowly reach out toward your toes, gently moving your upper torso forward over your legs. Your neck should relax as your head drops forward.

> ### TRAINING TIP
>
> If you find it difficult to keep your shoulders back and your back straight in the hamstring stretch, try one of these modifications:
>
> - Fold a blanket or a towel a few times and sit on the edge of it so that your rear end is slightly elevated.
>
> - If you're still uncomfortable, sit with your back against a wall or sturdy piece of furniture for support.

Go as far as you can *while keeping your back straight.* For many of us, that's not far at all — and that's OK! Stretching isn't a competition, and increasing your flexibility doesn't happen overnight. Enter the stretch gently, without fighting, forcing, or bouncing and with no agenda: instead embrace exactly where you are. Continue to breathe as you count to 10. You should feel the backs of your legs stretching.

After 10 seconds see if you can stretch a little farther, even if you add just another one-quarter inch to the stretch. Hold this new position for 10 seconds more. Remember, everything you do in Training for Life is relative to *your own* efforts, *your own* abilities, and *your own* body.

Now reach your hands high over your head again and go back again for one more set of seated hamstring stretches. Hold it a little longer — 15 seconds. Again balance your efforts to reach a little farther with an honest acceptance of what your body can comfortably do.

Note to Your Inner Coach

By definition, stretching is the opposite of contracting; when you stretch you are encouraging tight muscles to become open and more relaxed.

Talk about the perfect metaphor for today's WorkIn! Fighting the tightness by forcing muscles to stretch against their will is a losing proposition. It causes discomfort and injury, and ultimately you'll defeat the purpose, as your muscles will naturally pull back to protect themselves. A far better approach is to work *with* your muscles. Embrace your flexibility (or lack of it), stretch only when muscles are warm, and work in very small increments as you move compassionately beyond the inflexibility and resistance.

SWAN STRETCH

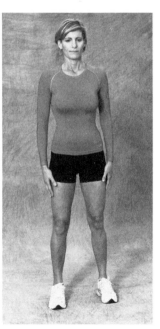

Stand tall, palms at your side. Open your arms and straighten them as you bring them up above you until your fingertips finally touch over your head. Before you dive forward, stretch up for a count of 5, feeling your arms lengthen and the muscles in your arms, shoulders, and upper back stretch out. Now bend forward at the waist, arms stretched out to the side in swan-dive position. You'll end up in a forward bend; relax your knees to reduce any stress on the lower back and in the backs of your legs.

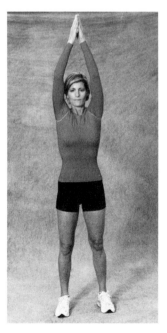

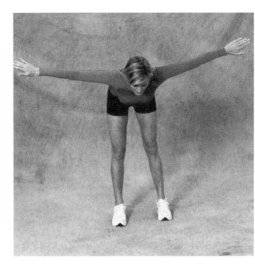

TRAINING TIP

Keep a slight bend in your knees (more if you need to). This will help you to eliminate excess tension in your hamstrings and your lower back.

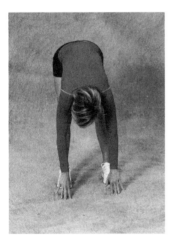

Hold the forward bend for a slow count of 10; then bend your knees even more and roll up very slowly, letting your head come up last. Keep your arms relaxed forward and then by your sides as you rise up, uncurling your spine, vertebra by vertebra. Once you're standing, reach your hands over your head again, stretching them up to the sky, and then slowly release them to your sides. Repeat this stretch again.

Embrace every aspect of your day today — especially the hard parts.

CHAPTER 16

Training Day Eight: Recovery

A Day of Rest

The chance to rest fully and completely doesn't come along very often. You may be lucky enough to stumble upon a day of rest, or you may have the foresight to plan one, meticulously organizing your week and hoping that nothing comes between you and your best-laid plans. You may even be granted one by someone who sees — more than you do — how much you need it.

Today I am taking that role: today's training day is a day of rest. I'd like to be clear: a "day of rest" is probably not what you think of when you think of a day off. This isn't a time to catch up on errands, old correspondence, or household projects — no matter how good you'd feel if you got those things off your list of things to do. Rest means freedom from exertion — all of it.

It has probably been a very long time since you last allowed yourself to fully rest. So long, in fact, that you may not remember how to do it; let me refresh your memory. First of all, tell your friends, family, and work associates that you're incommunicado — out of touch, gone fishing — and really *do* it. Arrange for a sitter. Turn off the phones, don't check your e-mail, do no shopping, no errands, no laundry — with no excuses. Instead take yourself to a peaceful spot, like the park or a beach, with a picnic, a blanket, and a bunch of magazines. Or stay home if that's what's more relaxing for you. Get lost in a good book or movie for a few hours. Put your feet up and read, take a long bath, or indulge yourself in a mid-afternoon nap. Don't do anything you are supposed to do or you don't want to do — just take it easy!

Now this *isn't* a break from training. You're always in training, even on a day of rest. So maintain your awareness and pay attention to the way you feel inside and out as you give resting your best shot. And this day of rest isn't a suggestion, it's a prescription.

You must learn how to take a break, not just from the hustle and bustle of your life but from the hustle and bustle of your *mind*.

Worry is exertion, obsession is exertion, projecting is exertion. So, to the best of your ability, allow yourself to be responsibility-free — even in thought.

Of course if you could just stop worrying and obsessing, you would have done it a long time ago; I understand that. Training, though, is our chance to practice changing the things that we want to be different about ourselves. In training we can isolate the habits that stress us out and keep us stuck and replace them with positive, prosperous, and healthful ones. With practice these new ways will become second nature for us. So train to let go of worry and stress by giving yourself the gift of a day of rest.

What if Day Eight falls on a workday? You'll just have to write yourself an IOU and cash it in at the first opportunity — before the breakdown, before the blowup, before an injury, an argument, or just a whole bunch of wasted, ineffective, low-level performance days. And even as you go off to work and about your other daily obligations on this prescribed day of rest, embrace the *concept* of rest and give yourself as much of it as you can. Don't neglect its importance — in your training or in your life.

WorkIn: Today is my day to rest, relax, and renew. Today I make way for my body, my mind, and my spirit to recharge.

Training for Life Meals

Make the same soup that you made on Day One, drinking the broth over the course of the day and eating a serving (one to two cups) of the vegetables for your evening meal. Be sure to also drink at least eight 8-ounce glasses of fresh spring water over the course of the day.

No WorkOut today; enjoy the rest!!!

CHAPTER 17

Training Day Nine: Strength

Train for the Unexpected

hen I started running marathons, I worked with a coach who'd take me out to run hills and flats, on concrete and sand and every other kind of terrain. We'd do long runs, mid-length distances, and short ones. In addition we'd swim, weight-train, and bike until my legs burned.

What Harry had me doing was cross training — the same thing the Philadelphia Eagles football team got so much attention for when they began including yoga as part of their standard training. Cross training means incorporating a variety of sports and conditioning activities into an athlete's training, not just those specific to her sport. It makes you stronger and more balanced, mentally and physically versatile, and prepared for whatever you may encounter during your event.

As my marathon drew closer, we eliminated everything but the runs, and I'd run longer and longer distances; that's called sport-specific training. But if you're Training for Life, as we are, cross training *is* sport-specific training.

The terrain of life is varied and unpredictable and requires many different activities at varying speeds and levels of intensity.

You're not a sprinter or a distance runner — you're both. You don't participate in one type of event, but *many.* So you must be many different types of athletes all rolled into one: a tireless employee, a compassionate spouse, the "world's greatest" parent, and a best friend.

And this is why in TFL we train for everything, alternating our focus between strength, endurance, and recovery. Sometimes our tasks call for short, powerful bursts of energy, like a wrestler: haul that kid out of the mud, into the bath, into pants, and into a car in fifteen minutes or less, just to get to your own birthday lunch. Or you may need the patience and stamina of an ultra-endurance runner to survive a day of back-to-back-to-back meetings and still be loving and attentive when you get home after enduring sixty minutes of traffic.

The training we do in Training for Life will give you the ability to handle whatever comes your way. You'll need it, too — *life is nothing if not unpredictable.*

Of course we must be physically capable of conquering any task we set ourselves to, but we must also be *mentally* prepared, so that we meet the unexpected with grace, the unplanned with ease, and the unforgiving with perseverance. Training for Life will give you a foundation so sound that you won't have to eat, drink, or self-destruct over a situation, even if it comes out of left field. Your training will give you inner and outer strength, so that you don't have to check out, freak out, or melt down. Prepared by your (cross) training, you'll be ready for everything!

I want to help you improve your state of mind, body, and being so that you feel, look, and live a lifestyle that says you're a winner, not just someone who finishes.

WorkIn: My training prepares me for everything — even the unexpected. Because of it I can tackle any challenge gracefully.

Training for Life Meals

Breakfast: three-quarters of a cup low-fat or nonfat yogurt or cottage cheese with one-third cup of berries and ten almonds.

Lunch: four ounces of sliced chicken or turkey breast on top of one cup of steamed or lightly sautéed vegetables or one cup of fresh green salad, with one slice of whole-grain bread.

Dinner: stir-fry. Toss two to four cups of fresh-cut veggies into a very hot wok or deep pan with one to two tablespoons of oil. Stir-fry for a few moments with a little salt and pepper, garlic, tamari, or white wine. Serve with three-quarters of a cup cooked whole-grain brown rice, basmati rice, millet, or quinoa.

Snack: two to four ounces of protein (tofu, chicken, or turkey slices).

Over the course of the day, drink eight 8-ounce glasses of water.

Strength WorkOut

STEP 1 (1–2 MINUTES):

Warm-up: Today we prepare for the unexpected, so you have 2 minutes, not our usual 5, to warm up. Do your best to relax as you walk, with abs engaged and shoulders down. Lift the crown of your head toward the sky as you go from YES 1 to YES 3 in 2 minutes.

STEP 2 (3–14 MINUTES):

Increase YES to 4 and walk for 3 minutes; then do the same at YES 5, 6, and 7, walking at each level for 3 minutes. Gear up and get ready for this intensified physical effort, even though it comes (unexpectedly) early in the WalkOut. Protect your body by keeping your awareness intact above all. Notice and manage your breathing, your stride, and your posture.

STEP 3 (15–17 MINUTES):

Reduce YES to 4 and walk for 3 minutes. These recovery periods (unpredictable in duration, as they will be in life!) train you to make the very most out of every moment that you find available for recovery.

Note to Your Inner Coach

Believing that you can do it is as important as any physical training that you do. This belief may require a leap of faith; you haven't ever done a Strength Training Day like this. But you have nine days of training under your belt, nine days of proving to yourself that you are capable of doing new, different, and demanding things.

All that previous training will enable your efforts today; don't hesitate to call on your mental conditioning — your focus, your ability to relax under pressure, and your newly improved confidence in yourself — to support you as we brave new ground. Don't let a little thing like surprise interfere with your progress!

STEP 4 (18–32 MINUTES):
Upper-Body WorkOut: Open Heart

Increase your pace and intensity to YES 5 for the next 15 minutes.

Bring your arms to field-goal position, bring your elbows together slowly in front of you, and touch them together (or as close as you can). Hold them there for 2 seconds and then open slowly for a count of 2. Keep the movement smooth and continuous for 8 sets of open heart over the course of the next 15 minutes, with 8 repetitions for Level I, 15 repetitions for Level II in each set.

STEP 5 (33–42 MINUTES):

Increase YES to 6 for 5 minutes, then to 7 for 5 minutes. With your arms by your sides now, use them to propel and sustain you at these higher levels of walking intensity.

STEP 6 (43–44 MINUTES):

You may have been expecting a recovery interval here, but there isn't going to be one. Why? Because recovery time just isn't that reliable. Muster up your strength and stay with me as we plunge forward.

Take it to YES 8 for 1 minute, then YES 9 for 1 minute: *hit it!*

Note to Your Inner Coach

What You Know Is More Powerful Than What You Don't

Sometimes we're on a clear path, but more often it's hard to predict exactly what will happen next. That's why it's so very important to train for the unexpected; it makes your mind more flexible, your body more powerful, and your spirit more resilient.

There will certainly be times — in your fitness regimen, and in life — when you feel uncertain, not knowing what's around the next corner. In these times it's helpful to concentrate on what you *do* know. You may not know how long it will take to get to the top of the hill, but you do know how to put one foot in front of the other and how to endure by calling on resources more powerful than your physical strength. Similarly, you may not know what's coming ahead during a WalkOut, but you can be sure that you will have the resources to handle it because it's based on your own effort scale.

Training for Life, and especially this training for the unknown, gives you a tremendous gift.

By the end of this program, you will know that you can always rely on yourself and the things you know.

When everything else feels uncertain or in flux, your commitment, focus, and efforts are rock solid, and in the end, that's *all* you need to know.

STEP 7 (45–49 MINUTES):

Reduce your pace, ease up your intensity, and relax your mind and body for 5 minutes at YES 5. This is by no means a chance to rest, but to recover efficiently, so you're amply prepared for what's coming next.

STEP 8 (50–59 MINUTES):

These intervals get more and more intense, but there's a silver lining: they also get shorter. Give me a banner effort and remember that you are training for the things that you *cannot* prepare for by being prepared for everything:

- Dial up YES to 6 for 4 minutes.
- Go to 7 for 3 minutes.
- Increase to 8 for 2 minutes.
- Finally, YES 9 for 1 minute.

STEP 9 (60–62 MINUTES):

Bring Your Effort Scale to 6 and take 3 minutes to moderate your breathing. This interval will show you that you don't need to slow your pace very much to recover.

STEP 10 (63–68 MINUTES):

Dial up YES to 7 for 3 minutes, 8 for 2 minutes, and 9 for 1 minute — AGAIN! Access the power that you have inside you; we've called on it before, so you know it's there.

STEP 11 (69–71 MINUTES):

Go back to YES 6 for 3 minutes. This is a good time for a mind-body check-in; make it quick, but make it count.

STEP 12
Level I (72–76 minutes):

Fantastic work. The hard part is over! Go to the R&R box below.

Level II (72–77 minutes):

Once again, dial up YES to 7 for 3 minutes, to 8 for 2 minutes, and to YES 9 for 1 minute. You are empowering yourself so that the unexpected will never throw you off balance.

STEP 13
Level II (78–80 minutes):

YES 7 for 3 minutes — believe it or not. Recovery is relative: when life throws you a curve, you may have to take your relief where you can find it.

STEP 14
Level II (81–83 minutes):

Back to 8 on YES for 2 minutes, then 9 for 1 minute. This is the proving ground. The work you are doing here makes you *better*.

STEP 15
Level II (84–88 minutes):

You crossed the finish line, you broke the tape — you did it! Fantastic work! Go to the R&R box below.

REST AND REFLECT

Take it easy on your way down, all the way to YES 1.

Be proud of your work today. You deserve to take full credit for your achievements in your training and in your life, especially on those days when things show up unexpectedly and pile up inconveniently. And although I certainly don't wish more of those days on you, I'm a realist, and I know they're coming.

TFL can help you conquer them with finesse and ease. You will feel more assured and more accomplished more of the time. Completing a training day like the one we've just finished must make you realize how capable you are. Keep it up, and you'll be a tough one to throw off balance — to say the least!

Stretch, Strengthen, and Tone (approximately 10 minutes)

TRICEPS DIPS (SEE PAGE 114)

Level I:
4 sets, 6 repetitions in each set.

Level II:
4 sets, 10 repetitions in each set.

LEG LIFTS (SEE PAGE 115)

Level I:
2 sets on each side, 10 reps in each set.

Level II:
2 sets on each side, 20 reps in each set.

ABCYCLE (SEE PAGE 132)

Level I:
4 sets, 6 reps on each leg per set.

Level II:
4 sets, 10 reps on each leg per set.

Have a great day — no matter what comes your way!

CHAPTER 18

Training Day Ten: Endurance

Body + Mind = Success!

One of the goals of this multitiered, mind-body training program is to **change your mind**, not just your body. You can't just change your body and expect your whole life to change, too, or expect to create a whole new you with the mind that's gotten you — and kept you — where you are right now. But you can condition your mind, the same way you condition your body, to change. And when you change your body and your mind, you can change your life, so that *all of you* becomes new, healthy, and totally fit.

Too often, our minds sabotage our efforts, instead of supporting them, but if you want to change your life, then your mind has to become your ally, instead of your enemy. Rather than providing you with excuses like "I'm too busy," "It's too early," or "It never works for long anyway," Training for Life will condition your mind to feed you more positive messages, like "I am going to train today, even though I'd love to stay in bed," and "Dinner's going to have to wait; I'm on the treadmill."

Your dreams *are* attainable. You can have your dream body, dream job, dream home, and anything else you can dream up. But you cannot attain those dreams if your mind is not on board. When I was running marathons, my coach Harry told me something that sticks with me to this day. He said, "When your legs get tired, use your arms." Of course, you don't run a marathon with your arms — but you *can* use them to help propel you forward and keep you going. Harry was telling me that I had to be willing to use everything I had to reach my goals, and I am telling you that your most powerful resource is your mind.

Your mind is a reservoir that you can dip into whenever you need to drum up some newfound excitement, focus in on a goal for inspiration, put things in perspective, or tap into a little extra discipline. This resource is easily renewable, infinitely powerful, and with you at all times. We will use it to ensure enduring success in weight loss, and in every other area of our lives.

So when your legs are tired, *use your mind.* When your arms are tired, *use your mind.* When you are restless, bored, weak, or feeling overwhelmed, *use your mind.* These are just temporary states; you have within you the power you need to pull you through to the winning side.

By the end of this fourteen-day period, you will have gained sufficient awareness to train safely, efficiently, wisely, and compassionately, according to your own desires and lifestyle goals. Excuses and sabotage will no longer create debate and struggle for you. You may want to stay in bed for another hour — who doesn't? But I think you'll agree that it's easy to leave those zzzs behind when doing so gets you that much closer to living your dreams, instead of just having them.

WorkIn: I condition my mind as well as my body for enduring results and total fitness success. My mind is an extraordinary resource, one that will help me change my body and my life for good.

Training for Life Meals

Breakfast: three-egg-white omelet with mushroom, tomato, spinach, onion. One-half grapefruit.

Lunch: one cup or can of soup and two cups of fresh salad sprinkled with dressing, with one-half cup cooked whole-grain rice.

Dinner: chili. Layer or mix together two cups of steamed vegetables (your choice), chopped in small chunks; four ounces of cooked, chopped, or ground chicken, turkey, or soy protein; and one-quarter cup of sugar-free tomato sauce. Eat with cucumber-and-tomato salad.

Snacks: one-half grapefruit; ten almonds.

Over the course of the day, drink eight 8-ounce glasses of water.

Endurance WorkOut

DAY TEN WALKOUT

STEP 1 (1–5 MINUTES):

Warm-up: Walk easily, slowly increasing intensity from 1 on YES to 3 in the first 5 minutes of your WalkOut.

While taking it easy you'll warm up, wake up, and begin generating mental and physical energy. This is where your work begins, so — forgive the pun — start off on the right foot. Walk tall, with poise, and lead with a powerful intention to succeed.

STEP 2 (6–20 MINUTES):

Walk 3 increasingly intense intervals of 5 minutes each, beginning with YES 4, then YES 5, and then YES 6. Use your mind to support your body's efforts as the work becomes more strenuous.

Note to Your Inner Coach

Today, more than any day of training, recognize the significance of the mind-body connection. As you train today, reinforce the importance of synergy between mind and body by repeating your WorkIn throughout your WalkOut: I condition my mind as well as my body for enduring results and total fitness success.

Your mind is your secret weapon. Training for Life focuses on developing this weapon. Use your mind to find inspiration when you feel disappointed and encouragement when you feel unmotivated. One way to do this is to remind yourself that the training you're doing will benefit the rest of your life, not just your body. This training is conditioning your mind and body so that you will live better, not just look better, for the rest of your life — now, *that* is success.

STEP 3 (21–25 MINUTES):

Dial down YES to 3 for an easy — but still steady — 5-minute recovery interval. Scan yourself — head to toe and inside and out — to make sure that both your physical posture and your mental attitude are where they need to be.

Note to Your Inner Coach

Stay with Me

Don't go away. It's tempting to zone out during recovery periods, but you must keep your "training head" so that you remain responsible, alert, and aware, even during these periods of low intensity. Stay focused, committed, and in touch with your desire to improve, even when you're in recovery. When you notice yourself spacing out, bring yourself back to your in-training state of heightened awareness as quickly as you can.

STEP 4 (26–35 MINUTES):
Walking Lunges

Slow down enough to begin your first set of walking lunges. Keep your stride strong as you step out with your knee over your front toes, dropping your back knee and bending your front leg just enough to create a right angle in front. Walk slowly enough so that you can keep the movement continuous throughout the walking-lunge interval. Walk 1 minute at YES 3 in between sets.

Level I:

5 sets of 5 on each leg.

Level II:

5 sets of 10 on each leg.

STEP 5 (36–51 MINUTES):

Do 4 intervals of 4 minutes each, starting with YES 4. Be sure to maintain a strong mental and physical posture as you increase to 5 for 4 minutes and then 6 for 4 minutes. Become even more diligent during the 4 minutes in your Power Zone at YES 7.

STEP 6 (52–56 MINUTES):

Dial YES back to 4 and walk your heart rate down. Spend these 5 minutes thinking about the enormous happiness and ease that a solid mind-body connection will bring you.

Note to Your Inner Coach

You Can't Change Your Body with the Mind That Got (and Keeps) You Here

"We can't solve problems by using the same kind of thinking we used when we created them."

— ALBERT EINSTEIN

I hated the sprinting my marathon coach made me do. I hated it. And I'm not proud of the way I behaved to get out of those training days — I pulled every trick, every excuse, every "emergency" out of my bag to get out of them.

I didn't — and don't — like doing things that I'm not good at, and I really don't like exposing my weaknesses to others. I believe that there's a powerfully useful component to pride, but there's a foolish part, too — and the part that prevented me from practicing a skill that would make me better and stronger was the foolish part. The big lesson of those sprinting sessions was the importance of *being teachable.* I needed to be open to taking direction and to doing things someone else's way, not just mine.

I have recognized this behavior in my students. One, in particular, is among the most powerful people in the movie industry, someone who can move millions of dollars and make or break a career with a phone call. But in his heart he's still the kid who got picked last for every team. When he first came to see me, he was overweight and out of shape; he had used the Mr. Hollywood part of his personality to charm, wheedle, cajole, or bully his various fitness trainers into doing things "his" way.

A lot of our work together was to get him to see that he was getting in his

> own way by refusing to do things someone else's way. He'd spent his whole adult life becoming the person who did the picking, someone who couldn't be crossed or corrected. But he was using that power against himself by sabotaging his training, allowing the foolish part of his pride to get in his way.
>
> You need your mind to be your ally, not to work against you. As you walk today, ask yourself if your own foolish pride or stubbornness isn't interfering with your ability to grow in some area of your life.

STEP 7 (57–71 MINUTES):

Do 3 escalating intervals of 5 minutes each. Begin at YES 4 for 5 minutes. Increase your walking speed and intensity to YES 5 for 5 minutes, to YES 6 for 5 minutes more, and pump your arms as you go, too.

STEP 8
Level I (72–76 minutes):

Excellent work! You can proceed to the R&R box opposite.

Level II (72–74 minutes):

For 3 minutes reduce YES to 4 and walk to recover.

STEP 9
Level II (75–79 minutes):
Walking Lunges

Over the next 5 minutes do 3 sets of 10 walking lunges on each side, with 1 minute of walking at YES 4 in between each set.

STEP 10
Level II (80–91 minutes):

Walk at YES 5 for 4 minutes, YES 6 for 4 minutes, then YES 7 for 4 minutes. Your combined mind-body effort is especially important now, when you're nearing the end of your training session. Staying focused and connected will help you work more efficiently and successfully.

REST AND REFLECT

Walk your pace down slowly, reducing intensity while keeping your posture as well as your attitude trained on success.

You've spent this time very productively focused on the finish line; now as you recover for the last time today, allow both your mind and body to relax. You're always at your most efficient when your body and mind are working together, whether you're striving to achieve a lofty goal or simply to recover and catch your breath. The efficient and dramatic results that come from this harmonious mind-body union are evidence of the mind-body connection at work. You are training to achieve this union and the harmony, freedom, and ease it brings.

So don't freak out when it happens! Suddenly, after you've spent years feeling like you've been fighting your way upstream, things will feel smooth and easily sustainable — and that can be unsettling! But you deserve every-thing you have worked for. So don't allow yourself to sabotage your efforts; instead, use the union of body and mind to stay on the road, deepen your practice, and further enrich your life.

STEP 11
Level II (92–96 minutes):
Move to R&R box above.

Stretch and Abs (approximately 10 minutes)

If you're wearing a WalkVest, remove it.

ABCYCLE (SEE PAGE 132)

Level I:
2 sets with 8 reps on each leg and a 30-second recovery period in between.

Level II:

3 sets of 12 repetitions on each leg and a 30-second recovery period in between.

SINGLE KNEE HUG (SEE PAGE 82)

Hold each leg — 2 times on each side — for 20 seconds.

ABCYCLE (SEE PAGE 132)

Level I:

2 sets of 8 each side.

Level II:

3 sets of 12 each side.

TOTAL RELEASE (SEE PAGE 133)

For 2 minutes at least.

TOWER

Sit up slowly, rise to your feet, and stand tall with your arms relaxed by your side and your legs and feet close together. Imagine that you are being lifted from the top of your head, while at the same time someone is gently pushing your shoulders down. Keep your chin level with the floor and stand still — but not stiff — for 30 seconds.

Then drop your chin for 10 seconds and allow the weight of your head to stretch out your spine. Slowly bring your head back up so that it sits lightly on your shoulders.

Enjoy a harmonious day.

CHAPTER 19

Training Day Eleven: Recovery

The Power to Rebound

We've talked about how even brief intervals of recovery can help you to comfortably and effectively endure during a WalkOut or over the course of a hectic day. But these recovery periods play another, very important role: they also fortify and assure your ability to **rebound**.

Let's face it: no one ever travels a road without hitting a bump. We're training for life, and that means that you're eventually going to make an unhealthy choice or one that you're just not very proud of. For you that may mean overdoing it with bread and butter at dinner or indulging too heartily at the office party. Maybe your effort during a WorkOut was weak or you didn't get it done at all.

That's OK. I forgive you — and I insist that you forgive yourself. If you stay on the road long enough, you are sure to encounter a number of hazards, as well as many great opportunities. You are being trained to recognize, and take full advantage of, the opportunities; similarly, this training conditions you *not* to let obstacles or mistakes become major setbacks. The Training for Life program provides you with what you need to bounce back if you falter, lose your way, or give in to unhealthy temptation.

From now on, see all interference as a learning experience and a chance to grow. In the past you may have let an eating mishap get the best of you, either by indulging in some "it doesn't matter anyway" eating or attacking yourself with guilt and self-recrimination. But we're going to take you far away from your old ways, and we need to do it fast. So no crying over spilled milk (or too much ice cream), no starvation diets, and no self-berating monologues. From here on forward, your power to swiftly rebound will stop you from getting caught in that self-destructive spiral.

So do not, I repeat *do not,* beat yourself up over yesterday's poor choices, and please don't try to compensate for them by eating only carrots the day after or swearing off bread for the rest of your life. That is not only a waste of energy but will throw you further off the Training for Life track. Instead continue as planned, making the "right" choices as you go forward. That's how you bounce back from a little "training malfunction," and every time you do it, you're participating in a very positive process: conquering your old habits, confirming your new desires, and *strengthening your ability to rebound.*

Each meal, each WorkOut, and each day will bring new choices and some new challenges, too. Dwell in the good, let go of the unfortunate, and keep moving steadily toward your healthier, happier life.

WorkIn: I will not let a setback send me back. Like any well-trained athlete, I have the ability to rebound quickly and to recover fully. No poor choice or obstacle will derail my progress toward a fit body and strong mind.

Training for Life Meals

Breakfast: one cup of cooked oatmeal with one piece of fruit.

Lunch: two cups of fresh, mixed green salad with two to four ounces of salmon, tuna, or chicken and one-quarter avocado, sprinkled with dressing.

Dinner: kebabs. Skewer two kebabs with two chunks of each: tomato, mushroom, onion and two pieces of either chicken, fish, or tofu. Serve with one-half cup cooked whole grains and two cups mixed green salad or cucumber-and-tomato salad (one half of a large or whole small cucumber and one small or one half of a large tomato sprinkled with dressing, rice wine, or balsamic vinegar).

Snack: ten almonds.

Over the course of the day, drink eight 8-ounce glasses of water.

Recovery WorkOut

DAY ELEVEN WALKOUT

STEP 1 (1–5 MINUTES):

Warm-up: Walk easily to warm up your body, gently and methodically moving from YES 1 to 3.

Walk tall throughout this recovery day, as you would on any other training day, and use today's WalkOut to rejuvenate your mind as well as your body.

STEP 2 (6–20 MINUTES):

For the next 15 minutes, you'll build your exercise intensity gently and slowly, in 3 increments of 5 minutes each.

First, increase the intensity of your efforts from YES 3 to YES 4, for 5 minutes. Savor your efforts as you move gently from the highest point in your Easy Zone (YES 3) to the lowest level of intensity in your Moderate Zone (YES 4).

Increase your efforts again, bringing YES to 5, and stay there for 5 minutes. Since in today's WalkOut you'll be moving a little more slowly and less intensely, take advantage of the opportunity to fine-tune your awareness. Pay close attention to your physical movements and notice your thoughts — whether positive or negative, peaceful or agitated — throughout. Practice calming yourself, whenever needed, by bringing the center of your attention to your breathing.

Move to YES 6 for the last 5 minutes. Here, at the top of your Moderate Training Zone, walk with a robust but relaxed stride.

STEP 3 (21–25 MINUTES):

Reduce your intensity, from YES 6 back to YES 3, and walk easily for 5 minutes.

STEP 4 (26–35 MINUTES): Upper-Body WorkOut: The Pyramid (see page 99)

Maintain YES at 4 for the next 10 minutes while adding this upper-body training to your walk. Do 5 sets of 8 reps for Level I; 6 sets of 12 reps for Level II. Make sure to take a short break (walking without arms for about 60 seconds) between sets.

STEP 5 (36–45 MINUTES):

Take YES to 5 and walk for the next 5 minutes. Your walking effort should feel *strong* but not the least bit stressful.

Then bring Your Effort Scale to 6 by pumping your arms and generating more intensity. Continue walking for 5 minutes more.

STEP 6 (46–50 MINUTES):

Dial down YES to 4 for the next 5 minutes and notice how your entire body experiences this recovery period; and don't forget to repeat your WorkIn.

STEP 7 (51–56 MINUTES):

Walk back up to YES 5 and then to YES 6, for 3 minutes each.

STEP 8
Level I (57–61 minutes):

Another WalkOut well done. Move on to 5 minutes of R&R.

TRAINING TIP

Your core is key. Contracting your abs supports your structural center and provides you with the postural integrity you need to safely train, especially when you're performing upper-body strength-and-toning work while walking. Your core should be active all the time, turning every walk into a core-conditioning body WalkOut.

A flat tummy isn't the only reason to work your core; having strength in this central area of the body gives a fundamental feeling of security and a sense of being centered and grounded in our bodies and in our lives.

TRAINING TIP

You can do these relaxation exercises while you walk; they feel amazing, especially after an upper-body exercise.

Shoulder rolls: Roll your shoulders backward and forward in exaggeratedly big circles, 3 to 6 times each.

Shoulder shrugs: Shrug your shoulders by bringing them as close to your ears as possible; then drop them down with a sigh and physical *release!*

Level II (57–68 minutes):
Stay at YES 6 for 3 minutes more, then recover at 4 for 1 minute; repeat this sequence (3 minutes at 6, 1 at 4) 3 times.

STEP 9
Level II (69–74 minutes):
It's your time now to proceed, proudly, to rest and reflect.

Chest opener: Clasp your hands behind you at your lower back (starting with your palms facing each other and interlocking your fingers) and squeeze your shoulder blades together behind you, bringing your elbows as straight and close together as possible.

I-love-myself hug: Wrap your arms around yourself in an enormous bear hug, grabbing your opposite shoulders, for a great upper-back, arm, and shoulder stretch.

Note to Your Inner Coach

Bouncing Back — Physically and Mentally

Awareness is of the utmost importance in making today's lesson a reality: after all, you must be aware of your old ways to stop and change them.

When you release your arms from the repetitious upper-body work, you can feel the transition as your physical body *rebounds*. After just a few seconds, your arms and shoulders have recovered, and you are ready to do another set. That is a powerful example of how your body rebounds. But what about your mind? How efficient are you at rebounding mentally? Can you pull yourself away from negative thoughts or self-destructive behavior, or do you find that you're more likely to get stuck in them?

My goal is for you to be able to get right back in line with your desire for improvement, even if you do act on a momentary lapse in judgment. This realignment is a Training for Life rebound, so keep Training for Life, and soon it will become second nature.

If you — like me — are the type of person who tends to get "stuck," then today's WorkIn will be very important for you. Just as your body gets fitter by repetitious conditioning, so will your ability to rebound improve by repeating your WorkIn for today.

REST AND REFLECT

Over the next 5 minutes or so, gradually decrease your intensity and energy output, all the way back to 1 on YES.

Today's training is specifically designed to enhance your ability to rebound and stay on the road; doing these internal and external exercises together will help you to become naturally adept at it, so that a little weariness won't sidetrack you, a little discouragement won't throw you off course, and a setback won't impede your forward progress.

So you stuck your hand into the kids' Halloween candy, ordered pizza when you shouldn't have, or slacked off on your exercise.

Making a mistake doesn't make you bad or worthless or a failure, and it doesn't take anything away from the good work that you have done to improve your body and your life.

We're all human. Don't let a mistake (or your reaction to it) set you off or send you back. Repeat your WorkIn and pledge to make better choices going forward. Think of these setbacks as switchbacks, those winding, roundabout roads that take you backward in the process of taking you forward.

Your heightened awareness is a powerfully useful tool; because of it, a light shines on all of your behavior. You'll no longer live an unexamined, unconscious life — or one filled with unintentionally ingested calories. But don't use this new awareness to abuse yourself. Paying attention to your behavior and forgiving it when necessary will prevent you from diving head-first into a negative spiral and contining to make the same mistakes over and over.

Training for Life works because it encourages you to be compassionate, not just vigilant. Rebound: acknowledge your misstep, forgive yourself, and go on with your productive day.

Stretch

If you're wearing a WalkVest, remove it.

CALF STRETCH (SEE PAGE 102)

Hold for 10 seconds and switch legs. Do 2 sets, held for 10 seconds on each side.

QUAD STRETCH (SEE PAGE 102)

Pick the quad stretch that was most comfortable for you. Hold for a count of 10. Slowly release and do the same thing on the other side for a total of 2 sets on each side.

CHEST STRETCH (SEE PAGE 104)

Hold for 10 seconds, release, and do the same on your other side, 2 sets on each side.

Have a great day — and if it doesn't feel great in any moment, don't worry: you have the power to rebound!

CHAPTER 20

Training Day Twelve: Strength

Opportunities vs. Obstacles: A Shift in Perspective

During our initial consultation Alison couldn't believe what she was hearing. "You've got to be kidding," she said. "I don't have that kind of time to work out! I have two demanding kids, one incredibly challenging job, and a husband who wants some attention, too. What you're asking for is impossible."

Cut to two years and fourteen days later. Alison's life has gotten even more complicated: she's been promoted to a position with even more responsibility, and her kids are now teens. But she's thirty pounds lighter, and her husband must be getting his fair share of love and attention, because he seems like a pretty happy guy. The only thing that's impossible now is getting Alison *not* to do her WorkOut on any given training day.

What happened? Two years ago Alison swore that there wasn't a single spare second in her schedule; now she finds an hour four or five times a week. Her job and her family life haven't changed — so what did?

Simple: **her perspective.**

Our lives are actually much more flexible than we are willing to allow; it's our thinking that's cast in concrete. If you make getting fit a priority, your life will accommodate it. Conversely, if you're not willing to put yourself — your weight, looks, health, and overall well-being — at the top of your long list of priorities, then nothing is going to change.

One of our goals with this program is to cause a fundamental shift in your perception. We've talked already about how much easier it is to get to the top of a hill if you see it not as an obstacle but as an opportunity to get stronger, to overcome your fears, and to break through your self-imposed limits. That kind of shift is possible in all areas of your life.

It's all about perspective: *that* is what shapes your life. When your perspective shifts, you find new freedom, more opportunity, and greater chances to grow and improve yourself without reservations or preconceived notions.

Change your perspective, and your whole world changes. Right now parent-child bonding in your family might mean a trip to the store after dinner for candy or ice-cream sundaes. Make the shift in perspective that I'm talking about and soon it will mean going on a bike ride, walking the dog together, or throwing a Frisbee around in the yard. Right now you may reward yourself with a chocolate bar or pastry; with a shift in perspective and in your priorities, you'll soon indulge yourself instead with a mani-cure or a new pair of jeans.

Today's Training for Life practice will reinforce some very important concepts for you: that your perspective shapes your life and that you have the ability to change that perspective, just as you can change your body, with daily conditioning exercises.

Alison once thought that she didn't have time to take care of herself; now she knows that *she can't afford not to.* Her outlook changed to support her efforts toward a better life, and her results reinforce that new outlook. Allow yourself to find the opportunity in every obstacle, and you'll see how quickly your life shifts — from closed to open, from difficult to fulfilling, and from overwhelming to brimming with opportunity. This is the training that will help you go from stuck to free.

WorkIn: My perspective shapes my life. I am opening my eyes and my mind to the opportunities ahead, including a brand-new me.

Training for Life Meals

Breakfast: one cup of puffed rice or Kashi cereal (no sugar added) with nonfat milk and one-half cup berries.

Lunch: bunless chicken, turkey, soy, or veggie burger, topped with lettuce and tomato, one-half tablespoon ketchup, and/or mustard. One cup of soup.

Dinner: stir-fry. Stir-fry two to three cups of fresh vegetables with four to six ounces of fish or chicken breast in one to two tablespoons of olive oil.

Snacks: ten almonds, one-half cup berries.

Over the course of the day, drink eight 8-ounce glasses of water.

Strength WorkOut

DAY TWELVE WALKOUT

STEP 1 (1–5 MINUTES):

Warm-up: Increase YES from 1 to 3. This is your time to notice — and tweak, if necessary — your perspective on today's WorkOut. These early moments help to determine how it will go, so ask yourself: How is your attitude today? Are you looking forward to the work ahead?

STEP 2 (6–17 MINUTES):

You'll do four 3-minute intervals of increasing intensity. And I'd like to remind you to stay focused on the level you're at; don't waste your energy by projecting ahead.

Increase YES to 4 for 3 minutes, 5 for 3 minutes, 6 for 3 minutes, and finally give me a powerful 7 on YES for 3 minutes more.

STEP 3 (18–20 MINUTES):

You have 3 minutes to recover at YES 4. This is a shorter recovery time than you're used to, and it would be natural to see this as an obstacle to your progress (and certainly to your comfort!). Shift your perspective so that you see it instead as an opportunity to become stronger. Less recovery time in training gets you ready for the rapid-recovery requirements of life.

I know that you can recover sufficiently in these 3 minutes if you make it your priority to do so. Focus in right away on reducing your effort intensity, relaxing your breathing, and softening your perspective.

STEP 4 (21–32 MINUTES):

Begin this sequence by walking at YES 5 for 3 minutes. You'll then walk for 3 minutes at YES 6, feeling the intensity increase as well as the heat that you are generating in your body. For the next 2 intervals, you'll be in your Power Zone. Use your mental power — not just your physical power — as you increase your pace to YES 7 for 3 minutes and then YES 8 for 3 minutes.

STEP 5 (33–35 MINUTES):

Again, you'll have a short recovery interval — walk 3 minutes at 4 on Your Effort Scale to recover.

STEP 6 (36–50 MINUTES):

Beginning with YES 5, walk for 5 minutes, moderately but power-fully, then go to YES 6 and walk for 4 minutes with a bit more intensity. At YES 7 you walk for 3 minutes, swinging your arms, and maintaining your posture mentally and physically. Next, you will walk at YES 8 for 2 minutes, using your powerful upper body to drive your pace. Make sure that your abs are engaged, your head is held high, and your shoulders are relaxed down. You have 1 minute left, and it's at YES 9 — what can I say but "hit it!"

STEP 7 (51–55 MINUTES):

Take 5 minutes to recover at YES 4; remember, recovery is always there when you need it (although not always when you *want* it!).

STEP 8 (56–64 MINUTES):

In this sequence you'll have 3 intervals of 2 minutes each with a 1-minute recovery interval in between.

Go to YES 7 for 2 minutes. Then recover at YES 5 for 1 minute. Repeat this sequence 3 times.

TRAINING TIP

When you're in your Power Zone — YES 7, 8, and 9 — your greatest ally isn't the power in your legs or your arms, but in your mind. That's why it's so important to see challenges as positive and useful, not as problems; use your inner strength and sense of perspective to aid and support everything you do on the outside.

Note to Your Inner Coach

A Compassionate WorkOut

As you've probably noticed you're working harder as this WorkOut progresses. If it seems unfair of me to ask that you give me *more* in the later stages of the WalkOut, then this will surely change your perspective: in fact, it's actually safer and more compassionate to train this way. Here's why: when your body has been active for 20 minutes or so, it's warm, flexible, and energized, and by this point in the WorkOut, your mind is alert, attentive, and engaged. So this is actually the best time to ask you for your strongest efforts. When you get tired, your recovery periods will help you regain your energy and strength, as well as your positive perspective.

All it takes to see a WorkOut as life enhancing and empowering rather than strenuous and exhausting (if you don't already) is a little adjustment in your perspective.

STEP 9 (65–67 MINUTES):

Decrease your efforts to 5 and walk for 3 minutes. Maintain a strong but relaxed stride, and walk with awareness.

STEP 10
Level I (68–72 minutes):

Beautiful work today — *hurray for you!* Go to the R&R box opposite.

Level II (68–77 minutes):

Go to YES 6 and walk for 4 minutes, YES 7 for 3 minutes, YES 8 for 2 minutes, and finish really strong today by walking at YES 9 for 1 last POWER minute!

STEP 11
Level II (78–80 minutes):

Maintain a moderately powerful pace at 5 on YES for 3 minutes. Walk with pride and purpose — you're in the homestretch, but you're not home yet.

STEP 12
Level II (81–85 minutes):
Go to R&R and revel in your accomplishments for a few minutes, but don't get stuck *there*.

REST AND REFLECT

What Do You Want?

Take 5 minutes to bring your heart rate and your breathing back to normal and make your way back to 1 on Your Effort Scale.

As you walk, I'd like you to think about *what you want.* Everyone has a vague sense of wanting "things to be better," but I'm a big believer in having tangible goals. When we really know what we want to achieve, then we can focus our efforts in that direction and determine the most efficient and effective way to proceed.

As your body cools down, I encourage you to think about your own personal goals. What do you want in, and from, your life? What does that look like, and feel like, to you? Don't censor yourself — include everything, large and small, pictures, sensations, feelings, or images.

Keep those desires close to your heart, and then ask yourself what the obstacles are that stand between your life today and the way you would like it to be. Is it possible that there's a shift in perspective that would allow you to see those obstacles as opportunities instead? If so, you're halfway there.

Stretch, Strengthen, and Tone (approximately 10 minutes)

If you're wearing a WalkVest, remove it.

WALKING LUNGES

Level I:
Walk 6 slow lunge strides on each side and then recover by walking 10 normal strides on each side. 3 sets.

Level II:

Do 10 walking lunges on each leg, with 10 steps (on each leg) in between. 4 sets.

TRICEPS DIPS (SEE PAGE 114)

1 set with legs extended. 1 set with knees bent.

   Note: If the legs-extended version is too stressful on your back or shoulders, do 2 with knees bent. If knees bent is not strenuous enough for you, do 2 with legs extended. Let your Inner Coach decide.

Level I:

8 repetitions in each set.

Level II:

12 repetitions in each set.

LEG LIFTS (SEE PAGE 115)

2 sets on each side.

Level I:

15 reps in each set.

Level II:

25 reps in each set.

ABCYCLE (SEE PAGE 132)

2 sets.

Level I:

8 reps on each leg per set.

Level II:

12 reps on each leg per set.

DAY TWELVE STRENGTH WORKOUT

CRUNCHES (SEE PAGE 83)

1 set.

Level I:
15 reps.

Level II:
30 reps.

SEATED HAMSTRING STRETCH (SEE PAGE 143)

Hold the stretch for 5 seconds, release, and repeat.

SWAN STRETCH (SEE PAGE 144)

Have an obstacle-free day — or at least try to see it that way!

CHAPTER 21

Training Day Thirteen: Endurance

Stay on the Road — Go All the Way!

In 1982 the world watched Julie Moss cross the Ironman finish line — a race that includes a 2.5-mile swim, a 100-plus-mile bike ride, and a 26.2-mile run — crawling on her hands and knees. It was an incredibly powerful moment and a testament to this athlete's spirit: she was trained to finish that race and determined to do it, no matter what it took.

Like Julie you are being trained to **go all the way,** and the only way to do that is **to stay on the road.** Your ability to do this reflects more of who you *are* than what you do. There will always be times when it's just plain hard to stay on the straight and narrow, to keep exercising, and to keep making the right food choices — but doing anything less is self-sabotage, pure and simple. You may feel bored with your WorkOuts at times, unhappy with the speed of your weight loss, or distracted for some other reason. Clearly, crossing the finish line won't always be easy, but it is enormously important that you do.

Training for Life helps protect you from the dangers of distraction and discouragement. You won't spiral out of control even when you're having a tough day or a hard week; you'll know that those are the times to renew your efforts, not to abandon them. We all experience plateaus and even setbacks; they're part of life, so you can bet that they'll be part of your training. It's the landslide effect that we have to watch for — a little disappointment can lead to "cheating eating" and excuses, and as we all know, that's when the self-recrimination begins. It's OK to stall or stumble, but you must keep moving forward toward your goals, and you must finish.

The only way to fail at Training for Life — or any of your goals, for that matter — is by quitting. That's what happened in your past, isn't it? Don't you dare give up this time. Feelings are fleeting, and overcoming them will leave you feeling empowered, unlike the lasting damage you do when you sabotage yourself. Your TFL training will provide you with the mental and physical exercises, motivation, and tools you need to get through the difficult times. It will (and I will) keep you focused, committed, and looking forward to meeting the new and improved you.

Until you can see this for yourself, you will have to take my word for it: staying on the road will take you to places that you have never been able to go before. I'll see you in the winner's circle!

WorkIn: I will stay on the road and go all the way. I will continue moving forward, every single day.

Training for Life Meals

Breakfast: one-half cup low-fat or nonfat yogurt or cottage cheese; one-half mango or papaya or one-half cup berries, and ten almonds.

Lunch: four ounces of salmon or chicken; two cups steamed or lightly sautéed veggies or two cups of fresh green salad with two to four tablespoons of dressing.

Dinner: bunless veggie, salmon, or turkey burger with sliced tomato, pickles, and lettuce with one-half tablespoon of ketchup and/or mustard and one cup lightly cooked (steamed or stir-fried) vegetables or soup.

Snacks: one fruit, one to two ounces of protein (salmon, chicken, or turkey).

Over the course of the day, drink eight 8-ounce glasses of water.

Endurance WorkOut

DAY THIRTEEN WALKOUT

STEP 1 (1–5 MINUTES):

Warm-up: Walk easily, going from 1 on Your Effort Scale to 3 in these first 5 minutes.

Use this time to gear up for the road ahead and know that no matter what I throw at you, you are going to stay on the road until you cross the finish line. That is what you are training for, and that is what you will do.

STEP 2 (6–25 MINUTES):

For the next 20 minutes, you'll walk with increasing intensity in 4 increments of 5 minutes each.

Take YES to 4 and walk for 5 minutes. Feel the warmth penetrate all of your muscles, then go to YES 5 for 5 minutes, increasing your intensity just a bit. Keep your focus and add the arms as you increase intensity to YES 6 for 5 minutes. Finally, marshal your efforts and take Your Effort Scale to 7 for a powerful 5-minute period.

Note to Your Inner Coach

What Can You Learn from How You Work Out?

These longer endurance intervals can be rich with useful information for you, if you're open to receiving it.

As frequently as possible, notice how your mental focus and physical energy fluctuate throughout the segment. Does your ability to concentrate increase over the time you spend working out or become more diffuse? Do you tend to go out with a lot of energy in the beginning, but lose steam toward the end? This is useful information: you'll know where you need to be more diligently alert and how physically conservative or aggressive you should be at the beginning of the next interval.

There's no judgment here, just information — and it's information about your training style that can be useful in your daily life as well, whether inside the gym or out. For instance, I'm someone whose focus intensifies as I go along. It takes me a little while to warm up, but I get more concentrated the longer I'm doing it. For me to be working at peak efficiency, I know that I have to set aside a block of time so that I'll have ample time to get into the activity. I also know that I need to minimize interruptions and distractions because I don't want to break stride once I've hit it — especially since it takes me some time to find my pace.

This information is very useful for me in all areas of my life. I know, for example, that it's hard for me to "squeeze in" a WorkOut; it takes too long for me to get warmed up and into it. And when asked to write this book, I knew immediately that I'd have to open up enough space in my work life so I could devote my full attention to it.

If you are paying enough attention and can recognize how you "work," you're demonstrating a level of focus and awareness that will contribute greatly to your ability to *stay on the road* and go all the way.

STEP 3 (26–30 MINUTES):

Turn the dial down on YES to 4 and walk your way back to recovery for the next 5 minutes. This recovery interval, like all of our recovery periods, provides us with the respite we need so that we are physically and mentally able to go all the way. Have a sense of that as you catch your breath and gear up for the next endurance interval.

Note to Your Inner Coach

Caution: Detour Ahead!

When Training for Life, you'll have everything you need to succeed, including motivational coaching, strength and endurance conditioning, and plenty of recovery. It's hard to think of a reason why you wouldn't stay on the road — but detours happen.

We're in the process of ridding you of your old beliefs and self-destructive habits, but they won't just vanish, and certainly not overnight. You will have to use your newfound awareness and the TFL exercises to overcome some of those latent urges. Soon you'll be more tuned in to your new voice, which will make opting for new, healthier choices easier. But you'll always need to stay alert, passionate, and vigilant, to the best of your ability. That level of attention and awareness will allow you to be more present in your life and to feel totally alive.

STEP 4 (31–45 MINUTES):

Repeat the sequence from step 2. This time you'll do 3 intervals of 5 minutes each, going from YES 5 to 6 to 7. Stay with it; go all the way. Practice your WorkIn by bringing it into your WorkOut right now.

STEP 5 (46–50 MINUTES):

Dial YES back down to 5 and walk your heart rate down. Again you'll be recovering in your Moderate Zone, this time at YES 5. Explore your body's ability to recover at different levels of intensity. Stay on the road; you're doing great work.

STEP 6 (51–60 MINUTES):

You'll do 2 intervals of 5 minutes each. Increase YES to 6 for 5 minutes and then again to YES 7 for 5 minutes. Staying fully present and "on the road" through longer interval periods in your Power Zone will require a most glorious concentration on your part, but I know that you have what it takes.

STEP 7 (61–65 MINUTES):

Reduce your effort slightly, to 6, and walk for 5 minutes. Don't let up — certainly don't "go away" or fall apart. Your mission is not just to hang in there but to stay strong. Contract your abs, throw your shoulders back, and walk proud.

STEP 8
Level I (66–70 minutes):

Excellent work! You can proceed to the R&R box below.

TRAINING TIP

Some days are easier than others. Some days my muscles feel fluid, my joints feel loose, and I feel blessed with the gift of good health and the ability to move easily. On those days my WalkOuts are over before I know it.

Other days I'm creaky and cranky. Every step feels like I'm walking through molasses, and it's everything I can do not to stop for some pancakes to go with it. Those are the days when it's hardest to stay on the road — and those are the tough times that we train for. Even with all the difficulty, it is enormously satisfying to complete a WalkOut on a day when nothing feels like it's coming easily. I know that staying on the road, even — or especially — when the going is tough, is the most important piece of the overall total fitness puzzle, and the feeling of accomplishment I get is magnificent.

Level II (66–70 minutes):

Dial YES up to 7 and walk for 5 minutes. Stay in it, and stay strong. Your body should feel warm, oxygenated, and gloriously alive. Take these 5 minutes to appreciate all these sensations and to fix your thoughts firmly on the finish line.

STEP 9
Level II (71–73 minutes):

Increase YES to 8 for 2 minutes and then to 9 for 1. Quitting is not an option, so make your effort as beautiful and pure as you possibly can as you bring this WalkOut home.

STEP 10
Level II (74–78 minutes):

Excellent work! Go to the R&R box below.

REST AND REFLECT

Driving into the Skid

Reduce YES slowly, from 6 to 5 to 4, all the way to 1.

Driving instructors always tell their students to drive *into* a skid. If you've ever hit one, you know that the advice is counterintuitive; you naturally want to wrestle with the wheel to regain control. But that's why you take driving lessons: to train yourself to do the right thing, even when it feels unnatural, so that your mind can override your instinct if the need arises.

That's how you should think of the endurance training we do in Training for Life. You will likely encounter some "dark nights" in the weeks, months, and years ahead, times when your weight loss seems stalled, you lack inspiration, or you struggle with a situation that makes your new healthy lifestyle difficult to maintain. In those moments the temptation will be very strong to give up and let it all go. You may not be planning to drop out completely, but more often than not, that is where those dark nights lead.

So when you find yourself facing one of these moments, don't do anything. Pause and take a moment to reflect on your training. Up until you met

---

me and Training for Life, you had been programmed to behave a certain way under certain conditions. But no more: we are changing those old patterns. With every WorkOut, and every repetition of a WorkIn, you condition yourself to trust, like, and believe in yourself. In so doing, you improve your ability to stay on the road. Train through the tough times, even when (or especially when) your faith feels weak, and that will ensure that you reach the light on the other side of the darkness every time.

Even if you just show up every day, it's a win. If you show up *and* dedicate your purest efforts to TFL, it's a major victory — and with that, I guarantee you the success and lasting results you're hoping for. There's no magic to this process; it simply requires that you stay on the road and go all the way.

Stretch and Abs (approximately 10 minutes)

Remove your WalkVest if you're wearing one.

ABCYCLE (SEE PAGE 132)

Level I:
4 sets of 6 reps on each leg and a 20-second recovery period in between.

Level II:
6 sets of 10 reps on each leg and a 20-second recovery period in between.

SINGLE KNEE HUG (SEE PAGE 82)

Hold for 10 to 20 seconds on each leg. Repeat 2 times.

TOTAL RELEASE (SEE PAGE 133)

Go all the way in your day today!

CHAPTER 22

Training Day Fourteen: Strength

Go Beyond Your Comfort Zone

We all strive for comfort in our lives. From how we live to the relationships we keep, we seek reassurance, support, and ease. When we find it we rarely stray too far away.

And that is how it should be — *up to a point.*

When we live our lives without awareness, comfort easily becomes complacency. Our habits, rituals, and familiar routines can provide us with security, camaraderie, and a safe harbor, but they can also imprison us. And when habits become deeply ingrained patterns, it can sometimes seem like change is impossible.

Believe it or not, being overweight is comfortable for you. And that's partly why you haven't been able to keep the weight off in the past; although you like the way you look and feel when you lose weight, it's also fundamentally uncomfortable for you — not just unfamiliar, but unsettling at your very core. At some level you still believe that being overweight (or underpaid, or single, or creatively unfulfilled) is all that you deserve. The thought of really changing is even more intolerable to you than staying where you are, or you would have been able to make these changes permanent a long time ago.

To bring about a healthy revolution in your life, you must break out of your comfort zone. If you want to look different, you have to do different things; if you want to feel different, you have to create different beliefs. That's what you've been doing in Training for Life over the last fourteen days. Every day, and in various ways, you have practiced letting go of your old, self-limiting thoughts; you are in the process of changing and eliminating your self-destructive patterns so that you will feel safe and at home in your new body. And the awareness conditioning that you are doing every day will allow you to be comfortable without becoming complacent.

When your fourteen days of training are up, you will have laid the groundwork for fundamental change, and you will have what you need to coach yourself going forward. Continue this inner and outer work, and you will keep letting go of self-destructive habits. You will be able to recognize your true desires — and attain them. Because of what you have set in motion, you will be able to continue moving forward bravely, beyond your comfort zone. Soon, getting exactly what you want will be all the comfort you need.

WorkIn: I will go beyond my comfort zone in order to improve my health, enhance my looks, and invigorate my life, even if it makes me uncomfortable for a while. My goal is to move forward in comfort, not to be still in complacency.

Training for Life Meals

Breakfast: one orange or one-half grapefruit and one or two soft-boiled or poached eggs, three tomato slices, and five cucumber slices. One piece of whole-grain bread.

Lunch: one cup or can of soup and one-half cup low-fat or nonfat cottage cheese with two cups of fresh salad and ten almonds.

Dinner: chili. Layer or mix together two cups of steamed vegetables chopped in small chunks; four ounces cooked, chopped, or ground chicken, turkey, or soy protein; and one-quarter cup sugar-free tomato sauce. Serve with cucumber-and-tomato salad and one-half cup cooked whole-grain rice.

Snacks: two grapefruits.

Over the course of the day, drink eight 8-ounce glasses of water.

Strength WorkOut

DAY FOURTEEN WALKOUT

STEP 1 (1–5 MINUTES):

Warm-up: After fourteen days you know what to do: walk easily, bringing Your Effort Scale from 1 to 3 as you prepare your body and mind for the work ahead.

STEP 2 (6–20 MINUTES):

There's no time like the present; although it may not feel comfortable, we're going from 3 on YES to 4 for 5 minutes. Then YES 6 for 4 minutes, YES 7 for 3 minutes, YES 8 for 2 minutes, and all the way to 9 for 1 minute.

STEP 3 (21–25 MINUTES):

Reduce intensity to YES 4 and walk easily, but with astute awareness, beautiful posture, and your "winner" intentions in place.

STEP 4 (26–34 MINUTES):

Increase your intensity, going all the way into your Power Zone. Walk at YES 7 for 2 minutes, then reduce intensity and recover on the road at 4 on YES for 1 minute. Do 3 sets.

Note to Your Inner Coach

Feel Like Pushing It?

Let's not just go beyond our comfort zone — *let's bust right out of it!*

At some point in your training, you will — if you haven't already — want to do *more* than what your coach asks from you. It's a wonderful feeling and a real hallmark of the transformation that's taking place in you. If going longer and harder and doing more is really what you need, then let your Inner Coach be your guide.

I'm asking you to push beyond your comfort zone today, but you must always stay within your safety zone. Transformation doesn't happen overnight, and you're much more likely to succeed if you train consistently and practice regularly, which is impossible if you're sidelined because you've overdone it. So don't hesitate to give a little extra — but only if you know you're still training smart and for the long haul.

STEP 5 (35–40 MINUTES):
Walking Lunge/Recovery Intervals
Over the course of the next 6 minutes, you'll do 5 sets of walking lunges with 30 to 60 seconds of walking at YES 4 in between sets.

Level I:
Each lunge set is 5 walking lunges on each leg.

Level II:
Each lunge set is 8 walking lunges per leg.

STEP 6 (41–51 MINUTES):
Walk at YES 5 for 4 minutes, YES 6 for 3 minutes, YES 7 for 2 minutes, YES 8 for 1 minute, and YES 9 for 1 minute. Walk tall and walk strong; be steady and be smart. Focus on your stride, your posture, your breathing, and your drive to succeed. Today is your day to push a little harder, work a little more diligently, and see if you are just a little bit stronger than you were yesterday. Go beyond your comfort zone, and you'll begin to see how comfortable your life can become.

STEP 7 (52–55 MINUTES):
Walk at YES 5 for 4 minutes. Collect your thoughts and physical composure as you recover and ready yourself to go again.

STEP 8 (56–65 MINUTES):
Dial up YES to 8 for 1 minute of powerful intensity, then down to 5 for 1 minute of recovery; do 5 sets.

STEP 9 (66–73 MINUTES):
Stay at YES 5 and walk for 2 minutes, then go to YES 6 for 2 minutes, YES 7 for 2 minutes, and YES 8 for 2 minutes. Comfortable or not, I know you'll do this!

Note to Your Inner Coach

Set the Bar Higher to Get Better

It's been a tough training day, but not too tough for you. Even working hard at very strenuous levels of intensity becomes comfortable after a while, so you must monitor your progress and drive yourself a little harder — as I have been doing for you in these past fourteen days — to make sure you continue to grow.

Driving yourself can be as simple as choosing a stronger, more experienced WalkOut buddy or playing against a more proficient tennis opponent once in a while. Listen to an advanced CD instead of a beginner one, increase the weight in your WalkVest, or add an extra half hour to your walk. Only your vigilant attention will keep complacency at bay, but your new awareness will allow you to determine the difference between complacency and comfort. Keep pushing yourself to do better — and, more important, to *be better*.

STEP 10
Level I (74–78 minutes):
Fabulous effort, wonderful work! It's on to R&R for you.

Level II (74–79 minutes):
Walking Lunge/Recovery Intervals
In the next 6 minutes, you'll do 5 more sets of walking lunges (8 lunge strides on each leg) with a 30- to 60-second walk at 5 on YES in between. Go on: push beyond your comfort zone safely, powerfully, and with pride.

STEP 11
Level II (80 – 84 minutes):
Remarkable work; you should be very proud! Go to R&R.

REST AND REFLECT

You Did It!!!

These 5 minutes are yours to savor — even to gloat over, if you wish — you've earned them.

Your WorkOuts and WorkIns should be paying off by now, on every inch of your body and in every area of your life. Your ability to take direction, to operate under new and unusual circumstances, and to bravely go where you have never gone before is worthy of a gold medal.

But it's what comes later that is your true reward. That's why we end these fourteen days with "Go Beyond Your Comfort Zone." It's time to leave the cocoon of day-by-day intensive coaching and direction and take on a little more responsibility and self-direction — now is your time to fly! But only, of course, if you feel ready. You can repeat these fourteen days as many times as you wish — most of my students do at least two times. You will know for yourself exactly where your needs lie because you have your Inner Coach and TFL to guide you.

Keep training, and the Training for Life practices will continue to enlighten and improve you, body and mind. I'm willing to bet that you'll be amazed by what you will discover about yourself, how easily you change, and how powerful you become.

Stretch, Strengthen, and Tone (approximately 10 minutes)

Remove your WalkVest if you're wearing one.

TRICEPS DIPS (SEE PAGE 114)

2 sets with legs extended; 2 sets with knees bent.

Level I:
8 repetitions in each set.

Level II:

12 repetitions in each set.

LEG LIFTS (SEE PAGE 115)

On your side. 2 sets on each side.

Level I:

10 reps in each set.

Level II:

15 reps in each set.

ABCYCLE (SEE PAGE 132)

4 sets.

Level I:

6 reps on each leg per set.

Level II:

10 reps on each leg per set.

SEATED HAMSTRING STRETCH (SEE PAGE 143)

SWAN STRETCH (SEE PAGE 145)

Do twice, holding the top stretch and the forward bend for 10 seconds each.

TRAINING TIP

Alternate these three exercises by doing 1 set of triceps, 1 set of leg lifts, and 1 set of abs in a circuit. When you work out this way, you won't need to recover between sets since you're training different muscle groups in each one. This keeps your heart rate up and intensifies your post-WalkOut training, and there isn't a better day to do that than today.

TRAINING TIP

Going beyond your comfort zone applies to stretching too. You need to push yourself a little bit to become more supple. But, as with your WorkOuts, *don't go too far.* The idea is to extend your reach, improve your posture, and enhance your level of fitness by gently pressing past the old ideas of what you are capable of. But if you go too far too fast, you can injure yourself — the exact opposite of what we're trying to accomplish. So go bravely but gently, just beyond what you feel is comfortable.

Congratulations, you are a Training for Lifer. I hope you live by this new moniker by staying with the TFL program and all of the commitments you have made and kept over the last fourteen days. You have taken significant steps on the path toward a new and improved body; enhanced health and fitness; and a finer, more fantastic life.

Stay on the road — and from here on out, go beyond.

PART THREE

LIVING YOUR TRAINING

CHAPTER 23

Now What? Life After Fourteen Days with Debbie Rocker

These fourteen days of coaching, intensive physical and mental conditioning, and your committed efforts have laid a solid foundation for your bright and beautiful future. Over the course of these fourteen days, you have learned the fundamentals of Training for Life and will take away with you a very powerful new set of skills. Now that this foundation is laid, you have some choices to make about how you want to proceed in the future; in this chapter I'll guide you through those decisions, but I suggest that you make them in close consultation with your Inner Coach.

Training for Life has three phases. You've just completed the fourteen-day program, which is the first of the three, and you may choose to do it again — and again, and again. I'd encourage you to repeat Phase I until you have attained your desired results and feel confident enough to move on to another phase of the program, one with less intensive coaching and training practices. You can always return to this most intensive phase of the program when you feel that you need this level of coaching and activity, even after you've progressed on to the other phases.

As you continue to train for life, you will become more independent and eager to flex your own coaching muscles. (For some people this happens immediately after the initial fourteen days.) But most people don't want to fly solo, so Training for Life also has two less rigorously structured subsequent phases, Phase II and Phase III.

Phase II is a two-week plan that features more food choices and more exercise options. It is designed to allow you to explore more options without throwing away your TFL training wheels. Again, although it is designed as a two-week program, many of my students find that they're most comfortable at this level and choose to stay here, either for a short period of time or indefinitely.

Phase III gives you a much less structured template for healthy living. It gives you a way for you to maintain the weight you've lost and to enjoy the freedom you've worked so hard for.

The great thing about the later phases of TFL is that fun counts as cardio. You'll see how Rollerblading, playing tennis, or coaching soccer for a couple of hours on a Saturday keeps you in terrific shape — and, maybe for the first time, you'll begin to feel the harmony between your daily life activities and your desire to stay fit.

In fact many of my students report that they've expanded their participation to include things they never thought they'd do. Christine had struggled with her weight her whole life, and her new job as an executive at a luxury foods company had made the problem even worse. When we first started working together, she was a full fifty pounds heavier than her tiny frame could comfortably carry. Unbeknownst to me, she spent the year after her first fourteen-day intensive in Phase II, walking with her WalkVest and my CDs. I heard from her again recently, when she sent me an e-mail with a picture of herself crossing the finish line at the Los Angeles Marathon. She's training to run San Diego now . . .

Christine credits her new slim body to Training for Life, but that's not all. In the same e-mail she told me that she had never before — even during her previous "skinny" periods — felt entitled or empowered enough to imagine that she could run a marathon or do anything like it. Now she feels whole and healthy, inside and out, and she's happy to live between Phase II and Phase III, guided by her Inner Coach.

You can do any phase of Training for Life at any time; that's the beauty of the system. If, for instance, you find that you have a hard time maintaining your results with the freedom allowed to you in Phase III, you may decide to stick with Phase II. If you enter an extremely busy and demanding period in your career or family life and have to scale back on exercise, the healthy and less demanding requirements of Phase III will keep you on track and still comfortably invested in your fitter life and body.

So any way you look at it, you're covered. This program can expand or contract to accommodate any change in your life; use it however you need to in order to stay totally fit for the rest of your life. Once you have successfully completed fourteen days with Debbie Rocker (no matter how many times you do it), there will never be a reason for you to go back to your self-limiting or self-defeating beliefs, your self-destructive or unconscious behaviors, or anything less than total fitness.

What Will I Eat in the Later Phases of TFL?

Keep your diet clean. Eat whole, organic, and fresh foods to the best of your ability. Steer clear of refined sugar, artificial (or unidentifiable) additives, preservatives, and sweeteners. You're going to be adding more items to your diet — but there's no reason ever to ingest junk.

Here are some things you will want to remember:

The less that's done to your food the better — and that means staying away from foods that are processed and prepackaged, like energy bars, microwavable meals, and fast foods, as well as those that have endured pasteurizing to sanitize them and the microwaving we do in the name of convenience. We really can do so much better for our bodies by not zapping the life out of our foods!

Dairy: I strongly recommend raw, unpasteurized dairy — raw milk, cheese, and butter. These products may be more difficult to find and more expensive — as all good, whole foods seem to be these days — but they are worth it. Why? Because they are natural, the way I ate them when I was young. My mother used to buy our milk straight from a local dairy, before it had been pasteurized, so that it contained all kinds of live bacteria — bacteria that can be supportive to our bodies. I'm grateful that I grew up on natural foods, thanks to Gramps and Mom. (And in case you're wondering, I didn't grow up on a farm in the heartland; I grew up in L.A.) I believe that these natural foods gave me a foundation that has stood me in good stead, despite later years of self-destructive behavior and poor nutrition. We must fortify our systems with the most natural foods possible to build a strong immune system and to sustain a youthful, healthy appearance.

Meat and Eggs: I choose, fertile, organic, and free-range eggs because they have not been heated or unnaturally processed, and they come from chickens that live in the healthiest, most natural environment. I also eat antibiotic- and hormone-free meat from organic, naturally raised animals. Crowded caging of any animal is unhealthy for the animal and for you, and it is something that I am morally opposed to. Many egg and meat producers do not follow compassionate or natural farming practices; I support the ones that do.

Fruits and Vegetables: All fruits and vegetables are OK in the later phases of Training for Life, so by all means add yams, potatoes, and corn back into your diet, but only two to three times a week, combined. All these foods should be fresh — no creamed corn, no French fries.

Wheat: When it comes to wheat, less is more. I do eat wheat, and certainly you will too — it's hard to avoid! But since it's in virtually everything, I do suggest that you try to reduce the amount of wheat you eat and vary your grain products to include millet, rice, spelt, and quinoa grains in breads, cereals, and pastas.

Read the ingredient panels! Remember, unless that package of rice pasta says wheat free, there's a good chance that there is wheat in there, even if other vegetables and grains are mentioned.

Desserts: Just because you treat yourself to something sweet every once in a while doesn't mean that you have to eat junk. If you do opt for dessert, choose something with fresh, whole ingredients. Whether it's pie, cake, cookies, or ice cream, don't blow it on nonfat, dairy-free, sugar-free junk; eat desserts made with real milk, butter, eggs, and fruit. Sweets should be only a very small percentage of your diet; opting for the fake stuff is actually less healthy and gives people license to overindulge. That's not something you want to do, no matter what you are eating.

As long as you don't feel compelled to eat dessert every time you go out or go to a party and have it only once or twice a week, you'll be fine — in fact, you'll be great! But if you can't eat dessert now and again without spiraling into a self-destructive binge, then don't eat it at all. Really, think about the trade-off — your sanity and lean physique versus fighting with a chocolate-chip cookie? Forget it — take dessert out of your diet and the subject off the table. (This is true, by the way, about anything you feel obsessed with or "addicted" to.) When you eliminate these foods, what you'll get in return is pure freedom.

Your Inner Coach has got to be present for all of your food choices; stay aware of your decisions and how they make you feel before, during, and after. And no use crying over spilled milk or poor choices — just decide to make better ones the next time.

If you find that you're going through a period where making the right choices is harder than usual, "reel it in." When in doubt I go back to eating according to the TFL basic plan, and you always can, too.

What Will My WorkOuts Look Like?

Phase II

Phase II is a little less physically demanding than Phase I and allows you to improvise when it comes to your Recovery WorkOuts. This phase is perfect for those of you who already have an active life but still need some structure and regular guidance.

Strength WorkOuts: Do these as they are written in TFL Phase I, two times a week.

Endurance WorkOuts: Do the Endurance WalkOut only, two times a week, followed by five minutes of abdominal exercises. (You should be able to do three to five sets of ten reps each in five minutes.)

Recovery WorkOuts: Three times a week, for a minimum of half an hour.

These aren't the recovery Workouts you've been doing over the last fourteen days. Just put on your sneakers and go for an easy half-hour walk at lunch. Walk with your dogs, your baby stroller, or your spouse (remember, the pace is easy — no showing off!); your pups will love it, and I'd bet your spouse could use it, too. Discover a neighborhood or nature walk you've never explored before. On these recovery days, one walk a day is good; two a day is better. Make sure you're moving at a steady and consistent pace for a minimum of half an hour a day.

Phase III

Phase III is perfect for people with a very demanding lifestyle. This WorkOut plan will keep you fit in a very efficient, five-day-a-week schedule.

Strength WorkOuts: Two Strength WalkOuts a week, as written in TFL Phase I, followed by:

- two sets of push-ups (eight to twelve reps each)
- two sets of triceps dips (eight to twelve reps each)
- two to four sets of walking lunges (ten reps on each leg)

Endurance WorkOuts: Two Endurance WalkOuts a week, as written in TFL Phase I, followed by five minutes of abdominal exercises. (You should be able to do three to five sets of ten reps each in five minutes.)

Recovery WorkOut: One Recovery WorkOut a week, consisting of thirty to sixty minutes of your favorite cardio exercise. Keep YES in your Easy-to-Moderate Zone, whether you're walking at the beach, dancing with your kids, pushing the stroller, or hiking.

With TFL you're never alone, even when you are on your own. You always have your TFL manual and CD to consult when questions arise, you hit a bump, or you just need a little extra guidance or motivation. As you settle into a comfortable, sustainable plan of exercising and a clean way of eating, you will probably spend less time listening to me and more time listening to your Inner Coach. Because you have been conditioned to be more honest with yourself and more self-aware, you will know when you need more Training for Life guidance and when you require less. No matter what, I am always here to support you in staying on the road as you travel this hopeful, healthful, and peaceful path — regardless of the obstacles (or should I say opportunities?) that you encounter.

CHAPTER 24

The Reward Is the Journey

Turn your attention within;

Don't memorize my words.

You have been turning from light to darkness

Since before you can remember,

So the roots of your subjective ideas are deep

And hard to uproot all at once.

This is why I temporarily use expedients

To take away your coarse perceptions.

— YANGSHAN, NINTH-CENTURY
ZEN MASTER

From a coach's perspective, there is no greater reward than being invited to work with a willing student like you. Like you, my reward is the journey. Working with you, coaching you, and seeking ways to reach you empower me as much as they do you. And I want to thank you for the opportunity to share in your success.

This book was designed to help you get back to where you deserve to be by universal right: in a state of happiness, healthiness, and freedom. The Training for Life practices are intended to help you condition your mind as well as your body, effectively and compassionately bringing the two back to where they belong — in harmony with each other and with the world outside. I did not give you anything new; you had it all when you came to TFL. All we did together was strip away the useless and destructive elements that had been hiding all of the good stuff inside you, like your strength, your hunger, and your desire to be better.

> **When you identify and remove the barriers to your dream body, you knock down the barricades that have prevented you from obtaining your dream life as well.**

Over the last fourteen days, you and I have performed a series of exercises designed to help you change your physical body; I hope those changes are noticeable and pleasing to you. You have also been given tools to develop your inner strength, your awareness, and the ability to differentiate between what is right for you and what is not. We have "trained your trainer" so that you can go from being a practicing student to your own best coach. We have awakened and developed your Inner Coach, which can now go on to support the choices you'll make for a more joyful, prosperous, and healthful life.

Over the last fourteen days, you have trained, like a true athlete, for the most important event that you will ever participate in: your life. You showed your willingness to change from the get-go by calling on a coach to help you. And you now have a new body, a new awareness, a dramatically improved attitude, and the TFL tools at your disposal. This is your new foundation, and it gives you the ability to sustain total fitness forever. It also gives you a springboard from which to launch new growth and to continue to evolve for the rest of your life.

You have proven, over the last two weeks, that with new ideas, new practices, and support you can rise above your old self-destructive behavior and self-limiting beliefs. You have stayed on the road, embraced resistance, and changed your perspective in the process of reconditioning your body and your mind. This fourteen-day finish line is a new beginning for you as well; as the conditioning continues, so can the transformation.

It's your time now, time to live and enjoy the life you have been training for, the one you have desired and always deserved. Grasp it with both hands and don't let it go. Use everything you now have — your TFL practices, your relationship with your Inner Coach, and me — to help you joyfully, powerfully, and healthfully *stay on the road.*

Blessings, peace, and happy trails forever.

Debbie

As a way of showing my appreciation for your effort and dedication to Training for Life, I'd like to offer you some of my favorite WalkOuts on CD if you decide to purchase a WALKVEST Training System. Simply go to the website (www.walkvest.com) and enter code TFL100 as you're checking out.

Walk in peace and good health,

Debbie

Training for Life WorkOuts at a Glance

TFL WorkOut Day One at a Glance

WorkIn: **I will stay *present* in the moment.**
(Repeat throughout the day 24 times.)

Strength WorkOut

WALKOUT

1–5 minutes: Walk easily, increasing intensity from **YES 1 to 3**.

6–14 minutes: Intensify your work as you walk at **YES 4** for 3 minutes, **YES 5** for 3 minutes, and then **YES 6** for a strong and steady 3 minutes more.

15–19 minutes: *Recover* by reducing intensity to **YES 4** and walking at a steady pace for 5 minutes.

20–25 minutes: Get back up to **YES 5** and walk a steady pace for 2 minutes, then increase to **YES 6** for 2 minutes, and then walk a very powerful stride at **YES 7** for 2 minutes.

26–30 minutes: Recover at **YES 5** for 5 minutes.

31–34 minutes: Increase to **YES 6** for 2 minutes, then **7** for 2 minutes.

35–36 minutes: Walk at **YES 8** for 1 minute, then **9** for 1 minute.

Level I:

37–41 minutes: Reduce YES slowly, going from **YES 9** to **YES 1** over these 5 minutes, and then on to stretching, strengthening, and toning.

Level II:

37–39 minutes: Recover quickly: 3 minutes at **YES 4**.

40–43 minutes: Increase from **YES 5 to 6** for 2 minutes, then hit and stay at **YES 7** for 2 minutes.

44–45 minutes: Continue at **YES 8** for 1 minute, **9** for 1 minute

46–50 minutes: Recover . . . at last! Walk **YES back to 1**.

Congratulations! You've done it! Celebrate your success by acknowledging your spirit and strength.

continued

Stretch, Strengthen, and Tone

FULL REST

Take a few moments of absolute peace and tranquility, body and mind.

PUSH-UPS

On your knees or full strength.

Level I:
3 sets of 5.
Level II:
3 sets of 8.

CHEST LIFT

Repeat 2 times.

SINGLE KNEE HUG

3 times on each leg.

CRUNCHES

Level I:
2 sets of 8.
Level II:
3 sets of 10.

CHEST LIFT

TRANQUILITY POSE

In these final few moments, embrace the new you.

Be mindful in every moment of your day today.

TFL WorkOut Day Two at a Glance

WorkIn: I am valuable.
(Repeat throughout the day 24 times.)

Endurance WorkOut

WALKOUT

1–5 minutes: Warm up by **increasing YES from 1 to 3 slowly.**

6–20 minutes: Start with **YES 4** for 5 minutes, then **YES 5** for 5 minutes, and then give me 5 minutes at **YES 6.**

21–25 minutes: Recover by walking at **YES 4** for 5 minutes

26–35 minutes: Walk for 4 minutes at **YES 5**, 3 minutes at **YES 6**, 2 minutes at **YES 7**, and then 1 powerful minute at **YES 8.**

36–40 minutes: Recover at **YES 5** for 5 minutes.

41–52 minutes: Go to **YES 6** for 5 minutes, **YES 7** for 4 minutes, then **YES 8** for 3 minutes. Be responsible, but make it memorable too.

53–57 minutes: Recover for 5 minutes at **YES 5.** You deserve it!

Level I:

58–62 minutes: Reduce **YES to 1**, then do your stretch and abs. *Great job!*

Level II:

58–60 minutes: Continue recovery at **YES 4** for 3 minutes.

61–68 minutes: Increase intensity to **YES 6** for 4 minutes; then, without a break, walk at **YES 7** for 4 minutes.

69–73 minutes: Reduce your pace, little by little, to **YES 1.** *Fantastic work!*

continued

Stretch and Abs

FULL REST

SINGLE KNEE HUG

2 times on each side.

CRUNCHES

Level I:
3 sets of 6.
Level II:
3 sets of 10.

TRANQUILITY POSE

Repeat 2 times.

Have a *priceless* day.

TFL WorkOut Day Three at a Glance

WorkIn: Recovery is a necessity, not a luxury.
(Repeat throughout the day 24 times.)

Recovery WorkOut

WALKOUT

1–5 minutes: Warm up by walking from **1 to 3 on Your Effort Scale**

6–20 minutes: Walk at **YES 4** for 5 minutes, followed by **YES 5** for 5 minutes, and then top it off with **YES 6** for 5 minutes.

21–25 minutes: Recover at **YES 4** for 5 minutes.

26–35 minutes:

The Pyramid while walking at **YES 4**.

Level I:

4 sets, of 6 repetitions each.

Level II:

4 sets, with 12 repetitions each.

36–40 minutes: Take **YES to 5** and walk with poise and purpose for 5 minutes.

41–43 minutes: Reduce **YES to 4** and walk for 3 minutes.

44–48 minutes: Take **YES to 1** over 5 luxuriously relaxed minutes.

continued

Stretch

Training Day Three: Recovery

CALF STRETCH

KNEELING QUAD STRETCH OR STANDING QUAD STRETCH

CHEST STRETCH

Have a very relaxed day.

TFL WorkOut Day Four at a Glance

WorkIn: My best effort is my greatest reward.
(Repeat throughout the day 24 times.)

Strength WorkOut

WALKOUT

1–5 minutes: Warm up, taking **YES** from 1 to 3.

6–15 minutes: Walk at **YES** 4 for 5 minutes, then **YES** 5 for 5 minutes.

16–20 minutes:

Open Heart while walking at **YES** 5.

Level I:

4 sets of 8 repetitions.

Level II:

4 sets of 15 repetitions.

21–28 minutes: It's time to intensify: walk at **YES** 6 for 4 minutes, then **YES** 7 for 4 minutes.

29–31 minutes: Hit **YES** 8 for 2 minutes, then **YES** 9 for 1 minute. It's time to really go for it.

32–36 minutes: Recover by walking at **YES** 5 for 5 minutes.

37–46 minutes: Increase to **YES** 6 for 4 minutes, **YES** 7 for 3 minutes, 8 for 2 minutes, and again for 1 brave minute at **YES** 9.

Level I:

47–51 minutes: Walk your heart rate down over these delicious 5 minutes and recover, bringing **YES** to 1.

Level II:

47–51 minutes: Reduce your intensity for 5 minutes at **5 on YES**.

52–61 minutes: **YES** 6 for 4 minutes, 7 for 3 minutes, 8 for 2 minutes, 1 minute at 9. Break the tape.

62–64 minutes: Walk at **YES** 7 for 3 minutes. Stay strong and alert.

65–69 minutes: Great job; take it slowly back to **1 on YES**.

continued

Stretch, Strengthen, and Tone

TRICEPS DIPS

Level I:

2 sets, 6 repetitions in each set.

Level II:

3 sets, 10 repetitions in each set.

LEG LIFTS

Level I:

2 sets on each side, 10 reps in each set.

Level II:

2 sets on each side, 20 reps in each set.

CRUNCHES

Level I:

3 sets of 8.

Level II:

3 sets of 12.

Let go of the results and enjoy the process.

TFL WorkOut Day Five at a Glance

WorkIn: My hunger is my desire to succeed.
(Repeat throughout the day 24 times.)

Endurance WorkOut

WALKOUT

1–5 minutes: Warm up to a great day ahead; take **YES 1** to **YES 3** over these first 5 minutes.

6–20 minutes: Walk at **YES 4** for 5 minutes, then **YES 5** for 5 minutes, then 6 for 5 minutes.

21–25 minutes: Slowly dial your intensity back to **YES 4**.

26–35 minutes:

Open Heart while walking at **YES 5**.

Level I:

4 sets of 10.

Level II:

4 sets of 20.

36–45 minutes: Rev it up a bit, going to **YES 6** for 5 minutes, then **YES 7** for 5 more.

46–50 minutes: Recover at **YES 4** for 5 minutes.

51–62 minutes: Increase intensity to **YES 5** for 4 minutes, then **YES 6** for 4, then hit **YES 7** and walk it out for 4 minutes more.

Level I:

63–67 minutes: Good job! Take 5 minutes to recover and bring **YES all the way back to 1.**

Level II:

63–65 minutes: **YES 4** for your 3 minutes of recovery.

66–77 minutes: Rev it up again: **YES 5** for 4 minutes, **YES 6** for 4 minutes, and **YES 7** for 4 powerful minutes.

78–80 minutes: Recover by dropping **YES to 6** and walk, steadily focused on breathing and form, for 3 minutes.

81–85 minutes: Yet again, well done! Over the next 5 minutes, take yourself all the way back to **YES 1**.

continued

Stretch and Abs

SNOW ANGEL

CRUNCHES

Level I:
3 sets of 8.
Level II:
3 sets of 10.

SNOW ANGEL

CRUNCHES

Level I:
3 sets of 8.
Level II:
3 sets of 10.

SNOW ANGEL

CHILD'S POSE

Have the day you hunger for!

TFL WorkOut Day Six at a Glance

WorkIn: I'd rather *be* better than feel better temporarily.
(Repeat throughout the day 24 times.)

Endurance WorkOut

WALKOUT

1–5 minutes: Move **YES** from **1 to 3** as you warm up.

6–25 minutes: Increase to **YES 4** in your next 5 minutes, graduate to **YES 5** for 5 minutes, **YES 6** for 5 more minutes, and then power it up at **YES 7** for 5 minutes more.

26–30 minutes: Dial down **YES** to 4 for a nice, steady recovery interval.

31–45 minutes: Rev it up: **YES 5** for 5 minutes, **YES 6** for 5 minutes, **YES 7** for 5 minutes more.

46–50 minutes: Recover now at **YES 5** for 5.

51–60 minutes: Give a little more: increase **YES to 6** for 5 minutes, and then to a powerful **YES 7** for 5 minutes.

61–65 minutes: Dial **YES back to 6** and walk for 5 minutes.

Level I:
66–70 minutes: Reduce to **YES 1** slowly. Excellent work!

Level II:
66–70 minutes: Dial **YES up to 7** and walk for 5 minutes.

71–73 minutes: Hit **YES 8** for 2 minutes and **YES 9** for 1 minute.

74–78 minutes: Reduce **YES to 1** slowly. You did it!

Stretch and Abs

CRUNCHES

Level I:
3 sets of 8.
Level II:
3 sets of 15.

continued

SINGLE KNEE HUG

Hold each leg for 10 to 20 seconds.

ABCYCLE

Level I:
2 sets of 8 on each side.
Level II:
3 sets of 12 on each side.

TOTAL RELEASE

Live your day in the right way.

WorkIn: Resistance is necessary, struggle is not.
(Repeat throughout the day 24 times.)

Strength WorkOut

WALKOUT

1–5 minutes: Over the next 5 minutes, increase **YES** from 1 to 3.

6–17 minutes: YES 4 for 4 minutes, **YES 5** for 4 minutes, and then **YES 6** for 4 powerful minutes more.

18–26 minutes: YES 7 for 2 minutes, then recover at **YES 5** for 1 minute. Repeat 3 times.

27–30 minutes: Recover at **YES 4** for 4 minutes.

31–40 minutes:

Walking Lunges while walking at **YES 5**. In between sets walk for 1 minute at **YES 5**.

Level I:

3 sets of 8 lunges on each side.

Level II:

5 sets of 10 lunges on each side.

41–46 minutes: Increase your pace and intensity to walk at **YES 5** for 2 minutes, **YES 6** for 2 minutes, and **YES 7** for 2 minutes.

47–50 minutes: Recover posture, poise, breathing, and focus at **YES 5** for 4 minutes.

51–59 minutes: YES to 6 for 2 minutes, then 1 minute of recovery at **YES 5**; back up to **YES 7** for 2 minutes, then recover at **YES 5** for 1 minute. Finally, dial **YES up to 8** for 2 minutes and recover for 1 minute at **YES 5**.

60–69 minutes: Here we go: Walk at **YES 5** for 4 minutes, **YES 6** for 3 minutes, **YES 7** for 2 minutes, and then **YES 8** for 1 minute of pure energy.

Level I:

70–74 minutes: Reduce intensity to **YES 1** over 5 minutes and breathe a sigh of relief.

Level II:

70–72 minutes: Recover at **YES 5** for 3 minutes. Stay alert.

73–82 minutes:

Walking Lunges while walking at **YES 5**. Do 5 sets of 10 lunges on each side, walking for a minute in between each set.

83–87 minutes: Walk **YES to 1** in 5.

continued

Stretch, Strengthen, and Tone

TRICEPS DIPS

2 sets with legs extended; 2 sets with knees bent.

Level I:

6 repetitions in each set.

Level II:

10 repetitions in each set.

PUSH-UPS

On your toes or on your knees.

Level I:

2 sets of 8.

Level II:

2 sets of 12.

LEG LIFTS

2 sets on each leg.

Level I:

10 reps in each set.

Level II:

20 reps in each set.

CRUNCHES

Level I:

3 sets of 10.

Level II:

3 sets of 15.

SEATED HAMSTRING STRETCH

SWAN STRETCH

Embrace every aspect of your day today — especially the hard parts.

TFL WorkOut Day Eight at a Glance

WorkIn: Today is my day to rest, relax, and renew.
(Repeat throughout the day 24 times.)

No WorkOut today; enjoy your well-earned rest.

TFL WorkOut Day Nine at a Glance

WorkIn: My training prepares me for everything — even the unexpected.
(Repeat throughout the day 24 times.)

Strength WorkOut

WALKOUT

1–2 minutes: Use 2 minutes to go from **YES 1** to **YES 3**.

3–14 minutes: Go to **YES 4** for 3 minutes, **YES 5** for 3 minutes, **6** for 3 minutes, and finally **YES 7** for 3 minutes.

15–17 minutes: Reduce intensity and recover with **YES at 4** for 3 minutes.

18–32 minutes:

Open Heart while walking at **YES 5** as you perform your open-heart intervals.

Level I:

8 sets with 8 repetitions each.

Level II:

8 sets with 15 repetitions each.

33–42 minutes: With your arms back at your sides, increase **YES to 6** for 5 minutes, then pump arms and walk at **YES 7** for 5 minutes.

43–44 minutes: Take it to **YES 8** for 1 minute, then **YES 9** for 1 minute: *hit it!*

45–49 minutes: Recover — mind and body — for 5 minutes at **YES 5**.

50–59 minutes:

· Dial up **YES to 6** for 4 minutes.
· Then **YES 7** for 3 minutes.
· Increase to a powerful **YES 8** for 2 minutes.
· Finally, hit it at **YES 9** for 1 minute.

60–62 minutes: Bring **Your Effort Scale to 6** for 3 minutes of recovery.

63–68 minutes: Here we go: dial **YES up to 7** for 3 minutes, to **8** for 2 minutes, and give me a grand effort at **9** for 1 minute.

69–71 minutes: Go back to **YES 6** for 3 minutes of recovery.

continued

Level I:

72–76 minutes: Slowly take **YES** back to 1.

Level II:

72–77 minutes: Walk **YES** back up to 7 for 3 minutes, then walk at **YES** 8 for 2 minutes, then take yourself proudly to **YES** 9 for 1 minute.

78–80 minutes: Recover at **YES** 7 for 3 minutes.

81–83 minutes: Back to 8 on **YES** for 2 minutes, then hit it hard one more time at **YES** 9 for 1 minute.

84–88 minutes: Take a well-deserved 5-minute recovery by walking all the way back to **YES** 1.

Stretch, Strengthen, and Tone

TRICEPS DIPS

Level I:

4 sets, 6 repetitions in each set.

Level II:

4 sets, 10 repetitions in each set.

LEG LIFTS

Level I:

2 sets on each side, 10 reps in each set.

Level II:

2 sets on each side, 20 reps in each set.

ABCYCLE

Level I:

4 sets, 6 reps on each leg per set.

Level II:

4 sets, 10 reps on each leg per set.

Have a great day — no matter what comes your way!

TFL WorkOut Day Ten at a Glance

WorkIn: I condition my mind as well as my body for enduring results and total fitness success.
(Repeat throughout the day 24 times.)

Endurance WorkOut

WALKOUT

1–5 minutes: Warm up, going from 1 on **YES** to 3.

6–20 minutes: Walk at **YES** 4 for 5 minutes, **YES** 5 for 5 minutes, and then **YES** 6 for 5 minutes.

21–25 minutes: Dial down **YES** to 3 for recovery.

26–35 minutes:

Walking Lunges while walking at **YES** 3 in between sets.

Level I:

5 sets of 5 on each leg.

Level II:

5 sets of 10 on each leg.

36–51 minutes: Walk at **YES** 4 for 4 minutes, stay steady at **YES** 5 for 4 minutes, stay strong at **YES** 6 for 4 minutes, and increase again to **YES** 7 for 4 minutes. Be powerfully diligent about form.

52–56 minutes: Dial **YES** back to 4 for 5 minutes.

57–71 minutes: Begin at **YES** 4 for 5 minutes, increase to **YES** 5 for 5 minutes, and add intensity to **YES** 6 for 5 minutes more.

Level I:

72–76 minutes: Take **YES** back to 1. You have done an EXCELLENT job!

Level II:

72–74 minutes: Reduce **YES** to 4 to recover for 3 minutes.

75–79 minutes:

Walking Lunges while walking at **YES** 4 in between sets.

80–91 minutes: **YES** 5 for 4 minutes, **YES** 6 for 4 minutes, then **YES** 7 for 4 minutes.

92–96 minutes: Bring **YES** back to 1 for a champion's recovery.

continued

Stretch and Abs

ABCYCLE

Level I:
2 sets with 8 reps on each leg.

Level II:
3 sets with 12 reps on each leg.

SINGLE KNEE HUG

ABCYCLE

Level I:
2 sets of 8 each side.
Level II:
3 sets of 12 each side.

TOTAL RELEASE

TOWER

Enjoy a harmonious day.

TFL WorkOut Day Eleven at a Glance

WorkIn: I will not let a setback send me back.
(Repeat throughout the day 24 times.)

Recovery WorkOut

WALKOUT

1–5 minutes: Warm up, walking from **1 on YES to 3.**

6–20 minutes: Rev up your efforts: start at **YES 4** for 5 minutes, then go to **YES 5** for 5, and then to **YES 6** for the last 5 minutes.

21–25 minutes: Reduce intensity from **YES 6 back to YES 3** and walk easily for 5 minutes.

26–35 minutes:

The Pyramid while maintaining **YES 4** throughout.

Level I:

5 sets of 8 reps.

Level II:

6 sets of 12 reps.

36–45 minutes: Walk at **YES 5** for 5 minutes and **YES 6** for 5 strong, stress-free minutes.

46–50 minutes: Dial down **YES to 4** for the next 5 minutes.

51–56 minutes: Walk back up to **YES 5** for 3 minutes, then **YES 6** for 3 minutes.

Level I:

57–61 minutes: Slowly reduce **YES to 1**, then move on to stretching.

Level II:

57–68 minutes: Walk another 3 minutes at **YES 6**, recover for 1 minute at **YES 4**; repeat sequence 3 times.

69–74 minutes: Reduce **YES slowly to 1** for your final recovery segment and then go on to stretching.

continued

Stretch

CALF STRETCH

QUAD STRETCH

CHEST STRETCH

Treasure the ability to rebound!

TFL WorkOut Day Twelve at a Glance

WorkIn: My perspective shapes my life.
(Repeat throughout the day 24 times.)

Strength WorkOut

WALKOUT

1–5 minutes: Increase **YES** from 1 to 3 for your warm-up.

6–17 minutes: Rev it up: begin with **YES** at 4 for 3 minutes, go to **YES 5** for 3 minutes, then on to a strong and steady **YES 6** for 3 minutes. Finally, give me a powerful **7 on YES** for 3 minutes more.

18–20 minutes: Recover for only 3 minutes at **YES 4**.

21–32 minutes: Rev it up again: **YES 5** for 3 minutes, **YES 6** for 3 minutes, up to **YES 7** for 3, and again to **YES 8** for 3.

33–35 minutes: Walk 3 minutes at **4 on Your Effort Scale** to recover.

36–50 minutes: **YES 5** for 5 minutes, **YES 6** for 4 minutes, **YES 7** for 3, 2 tough minutes at **YES 8**, and finally, 1 great minute at **YES 9** — all I can say is, "Hit it!"

51–55 minutes: You have 5 luxurious (but still focused) minutes to recover at **YES 4**.

56–64 minutes: Go all the way to **YES 7** for 2 minutes, then recover at **YES 5** for 1 minute. Repeat this sequence 3 times.

65–67 minutes: Decrease **Your Effort Scale to 5** and walk for 3 minutes.

Level I:

68–72 minutes: Take **YES to 1**; recover to stretching, strengthening, and toning.

Level II:

68–77 minutes: Walk with **YES** at 6 for 4 minutes, **YES 7** for 3 minutes, **YES 8** — mean it! — for 2 minutes, and finish really strong by walking at **YES 9** for 1 minute!

78–80 minutes: Enjoy walking at a brisk but relaxed **YES 5** for 3 minutes.

81–85 minutes: Finally, reduce your pace slowly to **YES 1**. Way to go!

Stretch, Strengthen, and Tone

WALKING LUNGES

Level I:

Walk 6 slow lunge strides on each side, followed by 10 normal walking strides on each side in between. Do 3 sets total.

Level II:

Walk 10 lunges on each leg, with 10 normal walking strides on each side in between. Do 4 sets.

TRICEPS DIPS

Do 2 sets total; 1 set with legs extended and 1 set with knees bent.

Level I:

8 repetitions in each set.

Level II:

12 repetitions in each set.

LEG LIFTS

Level I:

2 sets of 15 reps.

Level II:

2 sets of 25 reps.

ABCYCLE

Level I:

2 sets of 8 reps.

Level II:

2 sets of 12 reps.

CRUNCHES

Level I:

1 set of 15 reps.

Level II:

1 set of 30 reps.

SEATED HAMSTRING STRETCH

SWAN STRETCH

Have an obstacle-free day — remember, it's all about your perspective.

TFL WorkOut Day Thirteen at a Glance

WorkIn: I will stay on the road and go all the way.
(Repeat throughout the day 24 times.)

Endurance WorkOut

WALKOUT

1–5 minutes: Walk easily, going from 1 on **Your Effort Scale** to 3.

6–25 minutes: Take **YES to 4** and walk for 5 minutes, go to **YES 5** for 5 minutes, walk at **YES 6** for 5 minutes, and then at **YES 7** for 5 minutes more.

26–30 minutes: Turn the dial down to **YES 4** and take 5 minutes of recovery.

31–45 minutes: Increase the intensity to **YES 5** for 5 minutes, **YES 6** for 5 minutes, and again to **YES 7** for 5 minutes.

46–50 minutes: Walk **YES down to 5** for 5 minutes.

51–60 minutes: Increase to **YES 6** for 5 minutes, then to **YES 7** for 5 minutes, staying strong and steady throughout.

61–65 minutes: Reduce your effort just slightly and walk at **YES 6** for 5 minutes.

Level I:

66–70 minutes: Reduce **YES to 1** slowly, recover, and get ready for stretching and abdominal work.

Level II:

66–70 minutes: Dial **YES up to 7** and walk for 5 minutes.

71–73 minutes: Increase **YES to 8** for 2 minutes and then go to **YES 9** for 1.

74–78 minutes: Reduce **YES to 1** gently and get ready for stretching and abdominal work.

continued

Stretch and Abs

ABCYCLE

Level I:
4 sets of 6 reps on each leg and a 20-second recovery period in between.

Level II:
6 sets of 10 reps on each leg and a 20-second recovery period in between.

SINGLE KNEE HUG

TOTAL RELEASE

Go all the way in your day today!

WorkIn: **My goal is to move forward in comfort,
not to be still in complacency.**
(*Repeat throughout the day 24 times.*)

Strength WorkOut

WALKOUT

1–5 minutes: Walk easily, bringing **Your Effort Scale from 1 to 3.**

6–20 minutes: Go to **YES** 4 for 5 minutes, intensify to **YES** 6 for 4 minutes, go to **YES** 7 for 3 minutes, dig deeply at **8 on YES** for 2 minutes, and break through to a new level with **YES at 9** for 1 minute.

21–25 minutes: Reduce intensity to **YES** 4 and walk easily.

26–34 minutes: Walk at **YES** 7 for 2 minutes, then reduce intensity to **YES** 4 for 1 minute. Repeat this sequence 3 times.

35–40 minutes:

Walking Lunges maintaining **YES** 4 over the next 6 minutes, while you:

Level I:

Do 5 sets of 5 walking lunges on each leg, walking approximately 45 seconds in between sets.

Level II:

Do 5 sets of 8 walking lunges per leg on each leg, walking approximately 30 seconds in between sets.

41–51 minutes: Walk at **YES** 5 for 4 minutes, **YES** 6 for 3 minutes, intensify with **YES at** 7 for 2 minutes, **YES** 8 for 1 minute, and now go for it by hitting **YES** 9 for 1 minute.

52–55 minutes: Walk and recover at **YES** 5 for 4 minutes.

56–65 minutes: Dial up **YES to** 8 for 1 minute of intensity, then down to **YES** 5 for 1 minute of recovery. Do 5 sets of this sequence.

66–73 minutes: Continue walking at **YES** 5 for 2 minutes more, **YES** 6 for 2 minutes, **YES** 7 for 2 minutes, and give a true show of strength by increasing and staying at **YES** 8 for 2 minutes.

Level I:

74–78 minutes: Reduce your intensity slowly to **YES 1**. Your fantastic efforts have proven your commitment — recover now for 5 minutes.

Level II:

74–79 minutes

Walking Lunge/Recovery Intervals:

5 sets of walking lunges for you: 8 lunge strides on each leg with a 30- to 60-second walk at **YES 5** in between.

80–84 minutes: Reduce **YES to 1** and recover as you revel in your accomplishments.

Stretch, Strengthen, and Tone

TRICEPS DIPS

2 sets with legs extended; 2 sets with knees bent.

Level I:

8 repetitions in each set.

Level II:

12 repetitions in each set.

LEG LIFTS

Level I:

2 sets of 10 reps on each leg.

Level II:

2 sets of 15 reps on each leg.

ABCYCLE

Level I:

4 sets of 6 reps on each leg.

Level II:

4 sets of 10 reps on each leg.

SEATED HAMSTRING STRETCH

SWAN STRETCH

Stay on the road — and from here on out, go beyond.

Index

Day Thirteen, 178–84, 229–30
   dealing with "dark nights" in, 183–84
   learning from longer endurance intervals in,
     180–81
   learning to endure and, 129
   in Phases II and III, 199
enjoying the journey, 111
expectations, letting go of, 36–37

fatigue, 90
fear:
   of being left "without," 121
   of hunger, 122–23
feelings:
   acknowledging vs. acting on, 129
   of desire, discomfort with, 123
   eating and weight related to, 3, 9, 50, 117–18
fish, 54
flour, 53, 55
form, maintaining, 81, 111
fried foods, 53, 55
Full Rest, 78

getting out of your own way, 87–88
goals, perspective on obstacles between your
     life today and, 175
goal weight, 32, 34
Goethe, Johann Wolfgang von, 125
going all the way, 178–79
grains, 53, 54
grazing, 56–57
gum, 53, 55

habits, 8–9, 126
hamstring stretch, seated, 143–44
handling yourself with care, 85–86
heart rate, 47
Holtz, Lou, 36
hot baths, 44
Hubbard, Elbert, 126
hunger, 117–18
   fear of, 122–23
   for something that food cannot give, 3

I-love-myself hug, 167
injury, reducing potential for, 43, 44, 45, 81,
     100–101
Inner Coach, notes to
   acting your way to better thinking, 119–20
   allowing time to recover, 88
   avoiding "stuffing," 95
   believing that you can do it, 150
   bouncing back physically and mentally,
     167–68
   concentrating on what you know, 151–52
   driving yourself harder, 189
   eating appropriate amounts of food, 121
   embracing resistance and letting go of
     struggles, 137
   enjoying the journey, 111
   getting most out of recovery, 98
   getting out of your own way, 87–88
   high level of effort, 89
   keeping your "training head" during recovery
     periods, 158
   learning from longer endurance intervals,
     180–81
   learning to endure, 129
   letting go of results, 110, 111
   mental and emotional posture, 41
   mind-body check-in, 74
   overcoming latent self-destructive urges,
     181
   preventing foolish pride or stubbornness
     from interfering with training, 159–60
   pushing beyond comfort zone, 187
   recognizing and releasing tension and stress,
     139–40
   recognizing significance of mind-body
     connection, 157
   seeing things differently through contradic-
     tory terms, 97–98
   trusting yourself, 100–101
   working harder as WorkOut progresses, 174
   working with your muscles while stretching,
     144
   see also WorkIns

intensity:
    breathing and, 108
    effort scale and, *see* YES
    high level of, 89
    learning to endure and, 129

James, William, 7

kneeling quad stretch, 102–3

leg lifts, 115–16
listening to your body, 37–38
longer endurance intervals, learning from, 180–81
lunges, walking, 137–38
    training tip for, 140

Mayo Clinic, 17–18
meals:
    Day One (vegetable-broth cleanse), 57, 70–71
    Day Two, 86
    Day Three, 96
    Day Four, 106–7
    Day Five, 118
    Day Six, 127
    Day Seven, 136
    Day Eight (vegetable-broth cleanse), 147
    Day Nine, 149
    Day Ten, 156
    Day Eleven, 164
    Day Twelve, 171–72
    Day Thirteen, 179
    Day Fourteen, 189
    grazing and, 56–57
    guidelines for, 54
    see also diet
meats, 53, 54, 197
mental conditioning, 10–14
    believing that you can do it and, 150
    changing your perspective and, 170–71
    endurance conditioning and, 28

for enduring results and total fitness success, 155–56
    and letting foolish pride get in the way, 159–60
    rebounding and, 167–68
    for unexpected, 149
    see also Inner Coach, notes to; WorkIns
Mill, J. S., 33
mind, effecting changes to, 5, 10, 11–12
    see also Inner Coach, notes to; mental conditioning; WorkIns
mind-body check-in, 74, 101
mind-body connection, 5, 8
    acting your way to better thinking and, 119–20
    dissonance between body and mind and, 10
    harmonious union of body and mind and, 161
    recognizing significance of, 157
Moderate Zone, 48, 72–75
morning, working out in, 128
Moss, Julie, 178
multitasking, 68
muscle soreness, 43–44
    easing, 44, 45
muscle tension, 75, 101

New York Times, 57–58
numbers, preoccupation with, 32–35

obsessing, 147
obstacles, opportunities vs., 170–71, 175
open heart (upper-body WorkOut), 108–9
opportunities vs. obstacles, 170–71, 175
organic fruits and vegetables, 54
osteopenia, 20
osteoporosis, 20
overeating, 95, 121
overweight:
    as buffer to protect us from feeling, 9
    comfort zone and, 185
    as symptom of "dis-ease," 5–6

packaged foods, 55, 197
perspective, shift in, 170–71, 175